Helping people with
SEXUAL PROBLEMS
A PRACTICAL APPROACH FOR CLINICIANS

D1579382

Peter Trigwell MB ChB MMedSc MSc(PST) MRCPsych

Consultant in Liaison Psychiatry and
Psychosexual Medicine
Leeds General Infirmary, Leeds, UK

ELSEVIER
MOSBY

Edinburgh London New York Oxford Philadelphia St Louis Sydney Toronto 2005

ELSEVIER
MOSBY

Sections of this book have been modified from Trigwell, P. and Kirk, G. (2005) Psychosexual medicine for psychiatrists. In: Stein, G. and Wilkinson, G. (eds), *Seminars on General Adult Psychiatry*, second edition. Gaskell: London, in press.

Cover image kindly provided by Verdite African Art, USA.

ISBN 07234 3409-3

British Library Cataloguing in Publication Data
A catalogue record for this book is available from the British Library

Library of Congress Cataloging in Publication Data
A catalog record for this book is available from the Library of Congress

Notice
Knowledge and best practice in this field are constantly changing. As new research and experience broaden our knowledge, changes in practice, treatment and drug therapy may become necessary or appropriate. Readers are advised to check the most current information provided (i) on procedures featured or (ii) by the manufacturer of each product to be administered, to verify the recommended dose or formula, the method and duration of administration, and contraindications. It is the responsibility of the practitioner, relying on their own experience and knowledge of the patient, to make diagnoses, to determine dosages and the best treatment for each individual patient, and to take all appropriate safety precautions. To the fullest extent of the law, neither the Publisher nor the Author assumes any liability for any injury and/or damage to persons or property arising out or related to any use of the material contained in this book.

The Publisher

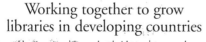

Working together to grow
libraries in developing countries

www.elsevier.com | www.bookaid.org | www.sabre.org

ELSEVIER   BOOK AID International   Sabre Foundation

The Publisher's policy is to use **paper manufactured from sustainable forests**

Printed in China

About the author

Dr Peter Trigwell, MB ChB MMedSc MSc(PST) MRCPsych, is Consultant in Liaison Psychiatry and Psychosexual Medicine at Leeds General Infirmary, Honorary Senior Clinical Lecturer at the University of Leeds and Founding Chair of the Leeds Sexual Dysfunction Special Interest Group (SDSIG).

The SDSIG is a multi-professional group with a membership which includes all those providing specific services for people with sexual problems, regardless of Trust or Sector. NHS services which are represented include primary care, urology, diabetology, gynaecology, genito-urinary medicine, psychiatry and endocrinology.

Since 1998 Dr Trigwell has been leading and developing a multidisciplinary psychosexual service in Leeds. This service treated over 1000 patients in the first 3 years of its existence and continues to expand in response to the increasing demand for specialist psychosexual help.

In addition to his Liaison Psychiatry interest, Dr Trigwell has carried out and published research in the field of sexual dysfunction, including the subject of sexual dysfunction in women with diabetes. His qualifications include a Masters degree in psychosexual therapy. He teaches on sexual dysfunction, amongst other subjects, and organizes regular study days on this subject for trainees from a broad range of medical specialties.

Contents

Foreword

Even in the 21st century, when sex is discussed in the media and in general much more openly than it was in the past, many people are experiencing sexual problems. Indeed, the numbers of patients presenting to doctors with such difficulties are increasing a great deal. Society's relentless emphasis on sex is raising expectations among people who may once have put up with less than satisfactory sex lives, and it is giving our patients the impression that everyone else apart from them is enjoying frequent and gloriously fulfilling sex.

As well as a growing demand from patients for help, there is a growing understanding among professionals that sexual difficulties may underlie recurring or otherwise inexplicable symptoms. An adult survivor of childhood sexual abuse, for example, may see many specialists and even go as far as surgical operations without anyone taking an adequate history of past or current sexual problems. At a less dramatic level, surveys have shown that women attending gynaecological clinics with the presenting problem of menorrhagia have a higher prevalence of sexual problems than a random sample of women.

Good medical practice involves developing a relationship of trust that will make it easy for the patient to reveal these very personal matters. It is common, however, for doctors to avoid taking a sexual history, not so much because of embarrassment but because of a feeling of helplessness about what to do if problems are identified. To most doctors, sex therapy is an obscure discipline far removed from the range of skills of the GP or even the gynaecologist. This is where this book can offer real help.

Textbooks on sexual problems can be disappointing. They may be weighty tomes full of psychological jargon or they may be unrealistic, set in a context unrecognizable to the busy clinician.

Dr Trigwell's book, by contrast, 'does exactly what it says on the tin' – it is a practical approach for the clinician who wants to help people with sexual problems. Providing such help requires empathy, common sense and the confidence that comes from training and experience, and it is the last of these that is lacking for most doctors.

Peter Trigwell is well supplied with empathy and common sense, and wears his considerable expertise lightly. Having worked with him for several years I have greatly appreciated his well-informed, down-to-earth approach and I believe our patients have also benefited. I am tempted to comment that only Peter could have written this book, which condenses a wealth of scholarship and experience into a readable volume of realistic advice.

Sex, more than most areas of human functioning, involves the mind, body and spirit working together. Helping people with sexual problems can be very challenging to our clinical skills, sometimes frustrating but often rewarding. Patients assume that doctors and some other healthcare professionals are trained to help them with their sexual problems, and this book is an ideal resource for those who want to live up to this expectation.

James Drife, MD FRCOG FRCPE FRCSE HonFCOGSA
Professor of Obstetrics and Gynaecology
University of Leeds, UK

Introduction

Sexual problems are common and important. Doctors and many other healthcare professionals, in a wide range of medical specialties, need to be able to assess, understand and offer effective help for such problems. Indeed, in several specialties, current Royal College guidance and curricula for training include a requirement for some specific training with regard to sexual health and sexual problems. The Royal Colleges with such specified requirements include those of physicians, general practitioners, obstetricians and gynaecologists, psychiatrists and nursing.

It is particularly important for trainees, as well as more senior doctors, to be able to demonstrate a working knowledge of the classification of sexual problems and dysfunction, which should include the organic/psychological interface of sexual dysfunction. They also need to be able to demonstrate a working knowledge of the management and treatment options available for sexual disorders, and to assess and formulate a management plan for people with sexual problems. In addition, some College requirements specify the need for a working knowledge of sexual identity disorders and paraphilias (Royal College of Psychiatrists, 2001).

Sexual problems carry with them a certain stigma. One result of this is that they are not easy problems to talk about, for either patients or professionals. Patients may not mention them until they have already developed a therapeutic relationship with their doctor or other member of the multidisciplinary team. They are also not likely to be volunteered without certain appropriate questions being asked. Indeed, it has long been known that a clinician who asks such questions as a usual part of taking a history will detect twice as many sexual problems as one who waits for the patient to raise the subject (Burnap and Golden, 1967).

Despite this, most doctors rarely take a detailed sexual history. When sexual problems are presented he or she may be unsure what to do to help. Most feel far from confident when it comes to making sense of, and helping people with, sexual problems.

It would not be appropriate for this book to try to teach the reader the entire topic of psychosexual medicine. Even if that was possible within a book of this size, most clinicians do not need to be experts in this field. Instead, this book aims to provide the reader with a basic understanding of sexual problems and a framework within which to be able to confidently assess, formulate and treat (or decide to refer on for treatment) their patients' sexual problems.

Sexual problems are generally subdivided into three areas (World Health Organization, 1992; American Psychiatric Association, 1994):
- Sexual dysfunction
- Gender identity disorders
- Paraphilias

This book concentrates upon *sexual dysfunction*. This is partly for reasons of brevity but is also in recognition of the prevalence and importance of problems with sexual functioning, and because they are presenting to doctors and other healthcare professionals with increasing frequency. Paraphilias and gender identity disorders are also covered, but relatively briefly and towards the end of the book (pages 83–89).

The clinical importance of sexual dysfunction

Prevalence and incidence

Difficulties with sex are rather more common than most people would suspect. Many men who come to clinic with erectile dysfunction as the presenting complaint are surprised, and sometimes relieved, to learn that over 10% of men in the general population (across the whole age range) suffer with erectile problems at any one time. Kinsey's surveys of sexual function in the mid 20th century found there to be an exponential rise in prevalence of 'more or less permanent erectile impotence' with increasing age (Kinsey *et al.*, 1948) (Table 1).

Rise in prevalence of erectile impotence with increasing age	
Age (years)	**Proportion with problem (%)**
20	0.1
30	0.8
40	1.9
50	6.7
70	27
75 plus	>50

TABLE 1. Rise in prevalence of erectile impotence with increasing age.

Another large but more recent study found that the prevalence of complete erectile dysfunction rises from 5% for men at 40 to 15% for men at 70 years of age (Feldman *et al.*, 1994).

Figures available from large scale surveys of other sexual dysfunctions include prevalence figures of 6% for premature ejaculation, 16% for female anorgasmia and 2.6% for female dyspareunia (Gebhard and Johnson, 1979).

Although such figures on classifiable sexual dysfunctions are available, perhaps what is really of clinical importance is sexual dissatisfaction. Just as with other areas of physical dysfunction, patients with sexual dysfunction (and their partners) vary with regard to the level of dissatisfaction reported. The relationship between these two areas is unclear. In a questionnaire study of 100 married couples in 1978, Frank *et al.* looked at the three areas of *sexual dysfunction, sexual difficulties* and *sexual dissatisfaction*. A higher proportion of women than men reported sexual difficulties (such as problems relaxing and a lack of interest). Around 60% of the women and 40% of the men had some degree of sexual dysfunction, and yet the figures for sexual dissatisfaction were 20% for the women and around 30% for the men. Apart from suggesting that sexual dysfunction is common, these figures give an indication that other aspects of the relationship may be more important in causing dissatisfaction, which may, in turn, be more likely to lead to people consulting healthcare professionals about their sexual problems (Frank *et al.*, 1978; Bancroft, 1989).

Considering how common sexual dysfunction is in the general population, and its association with both psychiatric and medical conditions, it is unsurprising that a high incidence of such problems has been found in studies carried out in a broad range of clinic populations and medical conditions, as shown in Table 2.

Despite the size of the problem of sexual dysfunction in clinic populations, little exists in the way of specialist services to help these people. With regard to psychogenic sexual dysfunction, psychiatrists sometimes find themselves in receipt of referrals from other medical colleagues trying to find psychosexual help for their patients. Where it has been possible to provide such services it has been found that, in addition to general practice, the majority of referrals come from urology, genito-urinary medicine, gynaecology and diabetology (as shown in Table 3).

Rates of sexual dysfunction in clinic populations/medical conditions	
Diabetes mellitus	Erectile dysfunction in 50% of men overall (25% in their 30s, 75% in their 60s) (McCulloch et al., 1980; Rubin and Babbott, 1958)
Family planning clinic (women)	Sexual problems in 12.5%. Of these, over 75% wanted help (Begg et al., 1976)
Genitourinary medicine clinic (STIs)	Sexual dysfunction in 25% of men and 29% of women (Catalan et al., 1981)
GP/urology/O&G	Sexual problems in an average of 15% (Burnap and Golden, 1967)
Gynaecology	17% with sexual dysfunction (anorgasmia) (Levine and Yost, 1976)
Mastectomy	No sexual activity in 33% after 1 year (Maguire et al., 1978)
Multiple sclerosis	Erectile dysfunction in 43–62% (Vas, 1978; Lilius et al., 1976)
Peripheral vascular disease	Erectile dysfunction in 40–50% (Wagner and Metz, 1981)
Psychiatric clinic	Sexual/marital problems in 12% (Swan and Wilson, 1979)
Stroke	50% do not resume sexual activity after stroke (Hawton, 1984)

TABLE 2. Rates of sexual dysfunction in clinic populations and medical conditions.

Referrals to a psychosexual service		
Referral source	**Number (n = 1000)**	**Percentage (%)**
General practice	529	52.9
Urology	209	20.9
Genito-urinary medicine	58	5.8
Gynaecology	56	5.6
Diabetology	30	3.0
Other (various med./surg.)	73	7.3
Unknown from database	45	4.5

TABLE 3. Referrals (the first 1000) to a psychosexual service, by referral source (Trigwell et al., 2004).

The effects of sexual dysfunction

In addition to the emotional distress caused, sexual dysfunctions have a range of clinically important effects. These are best considered under the following three headings:

i) EFFECTS UPON THE RELATIONSHIP

When sex is going well it is often just a small part of what is perceived as a good relationship. When sex becomes a problem, however, this can soon develop into a preoccupying issue for the person or couple involved. If not resolved, this will often lead to a deterioration in the general (non-sexual) parts of the relationship concerned. Repeated 'failures' of sexual functioning cause a whole range of negative emotions in both partners. These include embarrassment or humiliation, guilt, anger, hopelessness and low self-esteem. Along with a lack of positive reinforcement as a result of the sexual dysfunction, these negative emotions may lead to an avoidance of sex. If not addressed, major relationship problems may arise.

Problems with sex are often cited by people presenting in psychosexual clinics as the primary reason for the failure of previous relationships. By way of an example, a recent national UK survey found that 21% of men with erectile dysfunction reported that their relationship had broken down, and a further 9% that their relationship was in difficulty, as a result of their sexual problem (Impotence Association, 1997).

On occasions, of course, couples may adjust and 'normalize' with regard to the sexual problem, or even choose to enter into the relationship in the first place knowing that there is a serious sexual difficulty which may prevent sexual intercourse. In such cases it must be remembered that, for them, 'improving' sexual function may not necessarily be a welcome change and may even upset the current dynamics of their relationship. This illustrates the importance of considering each case individually and not seeing patients in isolation from their partner.

ii) EFFECTS UPON CHILDREN

Sexual problems can have a negative impact upon the children of a couple with such difficulties. This occurs as a result of their deleterious effects upon the relationship and their tendency to cause discord, so that divorce is a common outcome of relationship problems. In the early 1960s, almost 90% of children lived with two biological, married parents throughout their childhood and adolescence. By the late 1980s this figure had dropped to around 50% (Wadsworth, 1986). Recent research has shown that divorce has long-term risks for the children involved. These include more social, emotional, behavioural and academic problems. Hetherington and Stanley-Hagan, in an important paper in 1999, warned that the stresses encountered during and following divorce should not be minimized, and that when adverse outcomes do occur "they may be difficult to modify through educational or short-term therapeutic interventions" (Hetherington and Stanley-Hagan, 1999). In addition, another group in the same year reported a study which found a long-term correlation between parental divorce and depression and divorce in adulthood. The correlation between parental divorce and depression in adulthood was explained by the "…quality of parent–child and parental marital relations (in childhood), concurrent levels of stressful life events and social support…". To add to this concern, they also found a long-term association between parental divorce and the later experience of a divorce in adulthood, highlighting the risk of a repeating cycle of this problem (O'Connor *et al.*, 1999). Hetherington's paper also acknowledges the important fact that it seems to be parental discord rather than divorce or separation *per se* which is the damaging element (Hetherington and Stanley-Hagan, 1999).

iii) EFFECTS UPON THE INDIVIDUAL

Clinically significant anxiety states can be precipitated by sexual and relationship problems. Perhaps more commonly, depression may be caused in susceptible individuals. As a result of the lack of longitudinal studies it is difficult to be sure about the incidence of depressive disorders as a result of sexual dysfunction. What is clear, however, is that the two are linked. Sexual and relationship problems cause depression, but people who are depressed often also suffer with secondary sexual dysfunction. This may be an integral part of the depressive symptomatology, as in the case of loss of libido (Beck, 1967; Mathew and Weinman, 1982) or may be a consequence of antidepressant medication, causing impaired sexual arousal, erectile dysfunction or retarded ejaculation, as well as a loss of interest in some people (Balon *et al.*, 1993; Segraves, 1988). A comprehensive and regularly updated review of the effects (including side-effects) of psychotropic drugs is available in the *Psychotropic Drug Directory* (Bazire, 2001).

The fact that the common problem of sexual dysfunction can lead to such negative effects upon the couple, children and the individual serves to illustrate the importance of detecting and treating sexual problems effectively. Key to being able to do so is a clear understanding of basic 'normal' sexual functioning.

Understanding normal sexual functioning

For sex to work well, at least from a physiological perspective, four basic elements are necessary:

1. Intact **endocrine functioning** (i.e. normal levels of sex hormones). Several substances are important. Testosterone is the main sexual driver in both men and women, although with much lower levels in the latter. Sex hormone-binding globulin (SHBG) is also important, because much of the testosterone detectable in the bloodstream is bound to it. As a result of this, a high SHBG level can mean a low free (active) testosterone level. High prolactin levels can impair sexual drive in either sex, as can a raised oestradiol in women (although the level of oestradiol obviously varies depending upon the stage of the menstrual cycle).

2. Intact **vascular supply** to the genital areas. The external genitalia in both sexes are supplied by the internal pudendal artery, which is one of the terminal branches of the anterior trunk of the internal iliac artery (Snell, 1981).

3. Intact **neural supply** to the genital areas. Although this is an oversimplification, in essence genital arousal (erection in the male and vaginal/vulval engorgement and lubrication in the female) is mediated via parasympathetic fibres, and ejaculation/orgasm mainly via the sympathetic system. The parasympathetic supply runs from sacral outflow S2, 3 and 4, via the pelvic splanchnic nerves and the nervi erigentes to the genitalia. Sympathetic supply to the same area is via fibres from the thoracic and upper lumbar rami. The latter pass to the pelvic plexus (usually situated in front of the bifurcation of the abdominal aorta) and then on to the genitalia, either via discrete bundles or as a scattered network of fibres, sometimes within the pudendal nerve, although this distribution is quite variable (Bancroft, 1989).

4. Appropriate *cognitions* (i.e. sexually-stimulating thoughts/images). Although often not recognized by patients, and some healthcare professionals for that matter, this is of fundamental importance to normal sexual functioning. Problems with cognitions tend to be most important aetiologically in cases of psychogenic sexual dysfunction (as in the classic example of performance anxiety/spectatoring, as described later on pages 53–54). The reason sexual functioning suffers when thoughts are not sexually stimulating, and particularly when they are anxious or unpleasant thoughts, is that this impairs arousal as mediated via the autonomic nervous system.

In normal sexual functioning, the sexual response is generally considered to comprise the following stages:

- Drive and desire
- Arousal
- Plateau
- Orgasm
- Resolution

Schematic representations of male and female sexual response are shown in Figures 1 and 2, respectively. Both the male and female response curves may be divided into five stages, as described below, with the addition in the case of the male curve of the 'refractory period'. A large variety of female responses have been observed. The three shown in Figure 2 represent three common patterns ('A', 'B' and 'C'). 'A' is the cycle of a woman who, on that particular occasion, passes through all four stages, including orgasm. 'B' is that of a woman who becomes highly aroused but does not reach orgasm, and 'C' represents the rapid response to orgasm which might occur during masturbation. (See also Figure 6, page 39, for a new 'intimacy-based model of female sexual response' which has been proposed as a helpful alternative model regarding women who present with a lack or loss of sexual interest.)

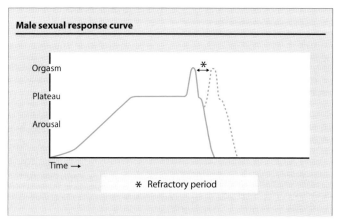

FIGURE 1. Male sexual response curve. From Hawton, K. (1985) *Sex Therapy: A Practical Guide*. Reprinted by permission of Oxford University Press.

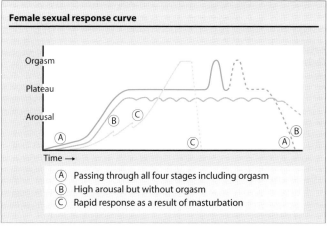

FIGURE 2. Female sexual response curve. From Hawton, K. (1985) *Sex Therapy: A Practical Guide*. Reprinted by permission of Oxford University Press.

Drive/desire

The initial stage of drive/desire may be considered to represent an individual's current level of interest in sex. Having said that, they are not identical concepts. Sexual **drive** is the perception of a need for sexual activity. That is, a basic human need which is largely biologically (hormonally) driven and not necessarily object- or person-specific. In contrast, sexual **desire** is the object-specific or person-specific correlate of that drive. In other words, one may have thoughts about sex in general and an urge towards sexual activity as a result of intact drive, but this tends to be experienced as an interest in and longing for sexual contact with a particular person, i.e. desire (Riley, 1999).

Arousal

Arousal is the stage during which more focused sexual thoughts and activity begin to occur. Perhaps the most noticeable correlate of the arousal stage is genital vascular engorgement, leading to penile erection in males and vulval/clitoral engorgement and vaginal lubrication in females. Research has confirmed the anatomical and physiological similarities between male and female genitalia. In basic terms, the glans penis is homologous with the clitoris, the shaft of the penis with the labia minora and the scrotum with the labia majora. There is no anatomical difference to suggest that the process of sexual arousal would vary to any great degree between the genitalia of men and women. In addition, the spinal centres of reflex control of the sex organs are similar and the involved afferent and efferent nerves entirely correspond (as described above). The response to tactile stimulation is also identical in both sexes, and from the physiological perspective erection in the male is identical with turgidity of the erectile tissue of the clitoris (Ellenberg, 1977). In both men and women, arousal builds via a complex mechanism of feedback loops, as illustrated by Bancroft in his 'psychosomatic circle of sex' (Figure 3).

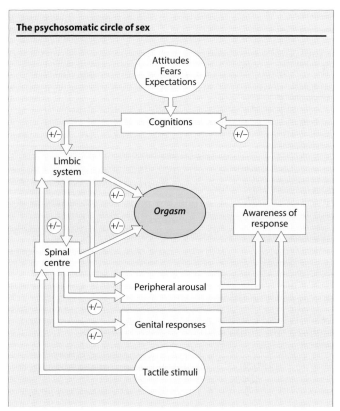

FIGURE 3. The psychosomatic circle of sex. Reproduced from Bancroft, J. (1989) *Human Sexuality and its Problems*, second edition. Copyright © 1989, with permission from Elsevier.

Plateau

During the plateau stage, the individual remains in a state of high sexual arousal. The duration of this stage is very variable between individuals, and within one individual on different occasions, and dependent upon circumstances. It may or may not eventually lead to orgasm.

Orgasm

Orgasm is difficult to define, which is probably why most texts avoid even attempting to do so. In his seminal and still outstanding textbook, Bancroft describes orgasm as "still largely a neurophysiological mystery, (which) involves both central processes in the brain and widespread peripheral effects experienced as acute increases in the intensity of erotic sensation and muscle contractions which are largely involuntary". It is these muscle contractions which produce ejaculation with emission of seminal fluid in men. The experience of ejaculation tends to occur at the same time as a more central sensation of orgasm, but the two are not identical and occur as different component parts of the overall experience of orgasm in the male. The process of ejaculation itself involves three main stages (Bancroft, 1989):

1. Pooling of seminal fluid in the bulbar urethra (emission may be perceived by the man as the 'moment of ejaculatory inevitability' or point of no return)
2. Tight closure of the bladder neck sphincter
3. Rhythmic contraction of the muscles of the penile base, causing expulsion of seminal fluid in 3–7 ejaculatory spurts at 0.8 second intervals

In women, the muscular contractions at orgasm are of the circum-vaginal/perineal muscles, also at 0.8 second intervals. Older texts tend to discriminate between two types of female orgasm. 'Vaginal orgasm' (i.e. due to vaginal penetration and penile thrusting only) was felt to be more powerful and in some way more mature than 'clitoral orgasm' (due to direct clitoral stimulation of some sort), which was viewed as inferior and immature in comparison. This notion is not now considered valid. There is, however, still a degree of controversy surrounding the idea of female ejaculation at the point of orgasm. This is connected with the concept of the Grafenberg or 'G' spot (Ladas *et al.*, 1982). In essence, it does seem that some women have vestigial prostatic tissue around the urethra, corresponding to a small area of increased sensitivity along the anterior vaginal wall. These women may emit a small amount of what is basically prostatic fluid from the urethra at orgasm, i.e. female ejaculation (Goldberg *et al.*, 1983).

Resolution

The final stage of the normal sexual response is resolution, when the body returns to its normal 'resting' state, with reduction in heart rate, respiration rate, skin flushing, genital engorgement and lubrication, back to their normal resting levels. This is an important time for physical and emotional closeness in a loving relationship – however, for some, especially if making love at the end of a long and busy day, sleep may follow rapidly. This can sometimes be a source of discontent for the sexual partner.

Refractory period

An addition to the five stages noted above is the refractory period in men. This is the period after orgasm during which it is not possible to experience further physiological genital arousal. It increases in duration with increasing age, so that in a teenager it may be only a few minutes, whereas it could extend to hours or even days in an elderly man (Hawton, 1985).

The general assumption is that with regard to any one particular episode of sexual activity these physiological stages occur in sequence, from 1 to 5. In fact, each stage is rather more independent than that. For example, ejaculation may occur without any sign of erection in a man with an erectile disorder, this being possible in view of the differences in neurological control of each of these stages.

Classifying sexual problems

The fact that sexual response tends to occur in the sequential stages mentioned above is reflected in the way sexual dysfunction is classified. Currently the most useful classificatory system is the fourth revision of the *Diagnostic and Statistical Manual of Mental Disorders*, produced by the American Psychiatric Association (DSM-IV, Table 4). In DSM-IV, 'sexual and gender identity disorders' are classified under three main headings:

- Sexual dysfunctions (the main focus of this book)
- Paraphilias (briefly covered on pages 83–87)
- Gender identity disorders (briefly covered on pages 88–89)

Classification of sexual dysfunctions

Specifiers:
- Lifelong/acquired type
- Generalized/situational type
- Due to psychological/combined factors

Sexual desire disorders
Hypoactive sexual desire disorder
Sexual aversion disorder

Sexual arousal disorder
Female sexual arousal disorder
Male erectile disorder

Orgasmic disorder
Female orgasmic disorder
Male orgasmic disorder
Premature ejaculation

Sexual pain disorder
Dyspareunia (not due to a general medical condition)
Vaginismus (not due to a general medical condition)

Classification of sexual dysfunctions (continued)

Sexual dysfunction due to a general medical condition (GMC)

Female hypoactive sexual disorder due to…(insert GMC)

Male hypoactive sexual disorder due to…

Male erectile disorder due to…

Female dyspareunia due to…

Male dyspareunia due to…

Other female sexual dysfunction due to…

Other male sexual dysfunction due to…

Substance-induced sexual dysfunction

Sexual dysfunction NOS

TABLE 4. Classification of sexual dysfunctions. Reprinted with permission from the *Diagnostic and Statistical Manual of Mental Disorders,* fourth edition. Copyright © 2000. American Psychiatric Association.

The basis for managing sexual dysfunction

The purpose of this book is to enable the doctor or other clinician to assess, understand and attempt to treat their patient's sexual problems, but also to be aware of their limits and when to refer on. After reading this book, a clinician should be able to make an assessment and attempt a formulation of their patient's sexual difficulties, paying attention to both organic and psychological aspects of aetiology. In what appear to be relatively straightforward cases, sensate focus and other techniques or relevant physical treatments should be used (as described in detail in this section), with referral on to specific services for difficult or complex cases, or any cases with which the clinician feels that he or she lacks the skills necessary to help the patient effectively.

A brief history of sex therapy

The history of Western approaches to understanding and dealing with sexual problems is briefly and schematically summarized in Figure 4. Before the enlightenment and advent of scientific (physiological and anatomical) explanations for bodily phenomena, common understanding was often in magical or supernatural terms. Corresponding remedies would also be in this vein (spells and charms), or involve seeking to redress the sin that was believed to have caused the dysfunction in the first place. A medical interest in sex and its disorders first developed in the late 19th century, followed by a more organized study of sex and sexual dysfunction in the 20th century. The work of William Masters and Virginia Johnson since the 1960s has had a particularly strong influence in the field of sex research and therapy, mainly through their description and use of a 'sensate

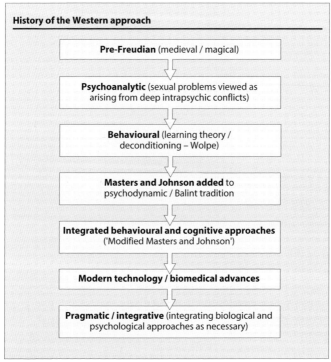

FIGURE 4. The history of Western approaches to understanding and dealing with sexual problems.

focus' approach as the basis for treating sexual problems (Masters and Johnson, 1966, 1970).

In the field of sex therapy, the psychoanalytical approach has largely been succeeded by the development of other psychological schools of thought, particularly cognitive behavioural. Behaviourism is based on Pavlovian and Skinnerian learning theory, so that behavioural treatments have developed using the principles of learning to change maladaptive behaviours, by weakening or eliminating maladaptive behaviours, whilst initiating and strengthening adaptive alternatives. More recently, the cognitive model put forward by Beck and others has taken further forward the development of organized cognitive behavioural forms of therapy. In essence, the cognitive model aims to address maladaptive thinking as the means by which to help with a person's problems, and is represented in Figure 5. Modern psychosexual therapy has developed out of these streams of thought into an integrated approach, which may combine psychodynamic, systemic and cognitive behavioural approaches to treatment but which, in the case of sexual dysfunction, increasingly uses the latter.

Over recent years we have also seen major advances in biomedical techniques and treatments for sexual dysfunction, such as the development of effective oral agents for the treatment of erectile dysfunction (e.g. sildenafil and tadalafil). There has been a parallel shift in social and cultural norms to accompany this development, particularly the heightened profile of erectile dysfunction and other male and female sexual problems in the media. The modern clinician will often need to use a combined, biopsychosocial approach in order to help their patients to successfully overcome their sexual problems.

Modern sex therapy (and how to approach it)

The approach to sex therapy outlined in the following sections of this book may broadly be described as a modified 'Masters and Johnson' cognitive behavioural approach. But what the technique is called, or how it is classified, is much less important than an understanding of how to use it to help people who are suffering with sexual dysfunction. The most important first steps are:
- Assessment
- Formulation and diagnosis
- Agreeing goals and treatment strategy

ASSESSMENT

The essential first stage in dealing with sexual dysfunction is a thorough assessment. The history should be taken in a chronological fashion; it is often most helpful to take background details first and to come on to the 'history of presenting complaint' (i.e. the sexual problem) thereafter, although it is obviously important to be flexible with regard to the order. In essence, what is required is a psychiatric-style history, with the following elements:

- Personal history (birth, development, childhood, schooling, work, finances)
- Social history (smoking, alcohol, drugs, forensic)
- Personality (relevant traits, pastimes, ways of coping with problems)
- Family history (members, relationships, familial conditions)
- Medical and psychiatric history (past and current)
- Current medications
- *Sexual history and functioning…*

The separate and detailed section on sexual history and functioning is of primary importance and should also be chronological in style. In eliciting the patient's sexual history, it is best to begin by finding out about the sources which may have contributed to the individual's attitudes towards sex and sexuality (e.g. religious beliefs, attitudes towards sex within the family, sex education, discussion with others about sex when growing up, masturbatory behaviour, etc.). The history of sexual activity with other people should follow, beginning with the first sexual experience that the patient had with another person, including detail as to the basic level of interest and functioning in the areas of arousal, plateau (sustained arousal) and orgasm. Each sexual experience/relationship should be covered in turn, concentrating upon these same areas of functioning. In other words, taking the sort of history which will facilitate an understanding of the development of the current problem and the nature of it, in accordance with the stages of sexual response as detailed earlier.

It is often necessary in this field to tolerate a degree of uncertainty with regard to the relative importance of physical and psychological factors. Having said that, one should attempt to decide whether the problem is primarily '*organic*' or '*psychogenic*'. Table 5 illustrates possible relevant information, using erectile dysfunction as the example.

When making a diagnosis, it is also important to consider whether the dysfunction is '*primary*' (having been present for the whole of the individual's sexual life) or '*secondary*' (having emerged after a period of normal sexual functioning).

Indicators of the aetiology of erectile dysfunction

	Organic	*Psychogenic*
Onset	Gradual	Sudden (may have a clear psychosocial precipitant)
Extent	Generalized (i.e. in any setting, alone or with a partner)	Situational (e.g. erectile dysfunction when with a partner but not when alone)
Early morning tumescence	Lack/loss of erections upon waking	Erections still occur upon waking
Ejaculation	May be normal (i.e. still occur despite no erection)	May be premature, normal or delayed
Life events	Often nil of note	Possibly relationship changes/life events or difficulties
Past medical history	Cardiovascular, neurological, endocrine, surgical or traumatic risk factors	Possibly no identified physical risk factors
Drugs and medications	Possible use of drugs/medications associated with sexual dysfunction	No use of drugs/medications associated with sexual dysfunction
Lifestyle	Possibly smoking, alcohol use (especially excessive or harmful use)	May be no lifestyle risk factors identified

TABLE 5. Indicators of the aetiology of erectile dysfunction. NB: This table is a summary/aide memoire. It is important to remember that organic and psychological factors can and often do co-exist.

It is best, whenever practicable, to interview the patient alone, their partner alone, and the couple together. This helps to ensure that as much relevant and meaningful information as possible is gathered. In taking a history in this way, however, it is very important to be clear with each individual whether there is any information which they do not wish to be disclosed when their partner is present, and to respect this request. On occasions this may cause a particular difficulty, such as in the specific case of ongoing infidelity about which one of the partners is unaware; this would generally be considered to make successful sex therapy with that particular couple impossible.

Physical examination and investigation

As a minimum, blood pressure measurement, random blood glucose and urine testing should be performed, along with appropriate physical examination (checking whether the external genitalia are normal and whether there are any signs of hormonal disturbance, or of excessive alcohol or drug use, etc.).

Where indicated by the history and examination, testosterone and SHBG (see page 9), luteinizing hormone, prolactin, urea and electrolytes, liver function tests, thyroid function tests and full blood count should be performed.

FORMULATION AND DIAGNOSIS

The aim of assessment is to generate a formulation of the patient or couple's problems. This means a description of the problem (i.e. diagnosis) plus an explanation in terms of the apparent aetiological factors (predisposing, precipitating and perpetuating). The formulation thus includes as clear an explanation as possible as to why this problem has arisen at this time for this individual or couple. Sometimes, when dealing with sexual dysfunction, the aetiology may not be immediately clear, particularly in relation to the relative importance of physical and psychological factors. It is important to set up treatment in a way that will allow ongoing assessment, and hopefully increased clarity with time. (See the description of 'sensate focus approach', pages 26–29.)

Sharing the formulation

This is a crucial stage in helping the patient or couple. The formulation is discussed and, hopefully, agreed upon. This is done so that both parties understand the nature of the problem, what is being proposed as the underlying cause, and what is being suggested as the plan for therapy. It is also an opportunity to give the couple hope and encourage a positive approach towards dealing with their problems.

AGREEING GOALS AND TREATMENT STRATEGY

A treatment plan is generated. This is done by considering which of the various treatment options is likely to be appropriate and acceptable, discussing this with the patient (and partner if he or she is to be part of the treatment strategy) and then implementing the treatment plan over a number of sessions. It is essential to agree goals with the patient or couple which reflect their needs and wishes, rather than basing the aims of therapy upon the therapist's own view of what would be a desirable outcome. Supervision is a key feature, as for any other psychological therapy.

Other treatment

Where necessary, ***physical treatments*** can be offered in conjunction with psychological work. This may mean co-working between specialties, for example in the case of patients under the care of both psychiatry and urology, or psychiatry and gynaecology, although prescribing oral agents should be within the capabilities of all doctors.

With regard to cases which, after initial assessment in primary care, are found to be organic in aetiology and to require specialist intervention, there is a range of possibilities for referral. Most urology services provide a specific service for male organic sexual dysfunction, which may be called the andrology service. Diabetes services also tend to provide clinics for assessment and treatment of male sexual dysfunction, mainly dealing with erectile difficulties. Clinicians working in genito-urinary medicine will see male or female patients with sexual dysfunction and gynaecology services deal with a lot of female patients with sexual problems, as do some dermatology services (especially with regard to vulval symptoms or pathology).

Local availability of services will vary but urology, diabetology, genito-urinary medicine, gynaecology and dermatology are the secondary services most likely to provide assessment and treatment for organic sexual dysfunction.

Specific physical treatments are discussed, where relevant to specific conditions, throughout this book.

General approach to sex therapy

Broadly speaking, sex therapy has three main components:
- Homework assignments (sensate focus approach)
- Dealing with blocks (cognitive 'troubleshooting')
- Education (an important element, to a variable extent, in every case)

This general approach is the core of sex therapy (Hawton, 1985). Specific techniques for specific conditions are also used, as described later, but on the background of this general approach to the therapy.

i) Homework assignments (sensate focus approach)

The sensate focus approach is used to provide a structure which allows couples to rebuild their sexual relationship over a period of time. It consists of pre-planned stages with clearly described homework assignments to carry out between sessions with the therapist. Although it is an effective basis for the treatment of most cases of sexual dysfunction, it must be remembered that sometimes it will not be suitable or effective, perhaps necessitating referral to a more specialist service.

Sensate focus is both a treatment and an ongoing assessment. In addition to helping the couple rebuild their sexual relationship, the aim is to allow further identification and clarification as to the specific factors which are maintaining the sexual dysfunction. There are four stages of sensate focus:

a) Non-genital sensate focus
b) Genital sensate focus

c) Vaginal containment
d) Vaginal containment with movement

a) NON-GENITAL SENSATE FOCUS

Following discussion of the formulation and an agreement to
pursue sex therapy, the couple are asked to agree to abstain from
penetrative sexual intercourse and to not touch each other's
genital areas (or the woman's breasts) until this becomes
appropriate in later stages of the approach. These elements of
sexual activity are temporarily 'banned' in order to remove the
sense of a need to 'perform' sexually, but it is obviously essential
for the couple to have sessions of time together in order to give
and receive physical (sensual if not yet sexual) pleasure. It is
suggested that they should have sessions lasting around 30
minutes, two or three times during the week, when they will
engage in touching and caressing. One partner will first explore
and caress the other's body (apart from the 'banned areas'), perhaps
using massage, stroking, kissing, etc. The partner who is receiving
this physical contact will give feedback to the 'active' partner. In
doing so they should begin each sentence with the word 'I', in
order to try to minimize the possibility of negative criticism. For
example, they may say "I really like what you were just doing" or
"I would prefer it if you did that more firmly", rather than
"you're not very good at that". After a period of time that suits
the couple (which should preferably be approximately half of the
session) they will swap roles. They should stop the session if they
become bored or if serious anxiety is provoked in either partner,
but otherwise the actual duration of the session would be
determined by what feels right for that particular couple.

These sessions improve trust and closeness, an awareness of what
each likes and dislikes, and may assist the therapist in clarifying
perpetuating factors with regard to difficulties that arise. The
couple should not proceed to the next stage of the programme
until they have been able to enjoy several sessions of successful

non-genital sensate focus. It is also very important to be clear that these sessions should be carried out in a private, warm and comfortable environment, with subdued lighting and with precautions to avoid being disturbed.

b) GENITAL SENSATE FOCUS

In this next stage of the programme the couple will be allowed to touch the genital and breast areas which were previously 'out of bounds'. It is important to avoid any misunderstandings, however, which might suggest to the couple that they should go straight to these areas; this stage should be **added** to the previous activity carried out during non-genital sensate focus. Penetrative sexual intercourse remains banned during this stage. Each partner should continue to focus upon the sensations being experienced, proceeding on to the more overtly sexual areas if that feels acceptable to them. They should not strive to become aroused or put any pressure upon each other to do so. In fact, a truly adult-to-adult agreement by the couple **not** yet to proceed to penetration should make physiological genital arousal much less relevant. Specific details regarding gentle touching and switching attention from one part of the body to another should be given by the therapist. It may be helpful to describe the genital touching, at least initially, as 'genital exploration', to distinguish it from behaviour specifically aimed at producing arousal. The couple should continue to feel relaxed and concentrate upon the giving and receiving of pleasure, and feedback should continue, as in the previous stage.

c) VAGINAL CONTAINMENT

The title of this stage sounds very clinical to some couples, so that the therapist may choose to use different words to describe it. In essence, however, this stage involves the gradual introduction of sexual intercourse whilst trying to minimize the anxiety which may be induced in some couples with regard to penetrative sex. This may be the case in men suffering premature ejaculation or erectile dysfunction, or women with the problem of vaginismus (described in more detail later). The couple should move on to this stage during a session of mutual pleasuring when they both feel relaxed and sexually aroused. Female superior is the most suitable position, with the male superior ('missionary') position not usually being recommended at this stage, as it increases the likelihood of ejaculation and is not a position in which a woman with sexual anxieties would feel in control. Once penetration has occurred the couple should remain still, concentrating upon pleasant genital sensations, although the man may move a little to stimulate himself if his erection begins to wane. Containment should last for whatever period of time the partners feel comfortable with, following which they should withdraw and continue pleasuring each other as previously described. Hawton suggests that vaginal containment should be repeated two or three times in any one session (Hawton, 1985).

d) VAGINAL CONTAINMENT WITH MOVEMENT

This is the final stage of sensate focus. It is generally most appropriate for the woman to move first, slowly initially but perhaps more vigorously with time to establish or re-establish full sexual intercourse. Thereafter, the therapist may suggest to the couple that they experiment with different positions, whilst remaining cognizant of their particular anxieties and any specific sexual activity which might always remain unacceptable for either of them.

ii) Dealing with blocks (cognitive 'troubleshooting')

Most couples encounter difficulties at some stage of the sensate focus approach. It is important to recognize such difficulties as a source of additional information regarding the aetiology of the couple's problems. When initiating sex therapy it is, therefore, helpful to discuss with the couple the need for them to return to clinic even if their homework assignments do not seem to go well. Difficulties can be positively reframed as providing useful information, and therefore increasing the likelihood of eventual success through therapy.

Minor blocks to therapy are very common, and include partners not initiating sessions due to feelings of embarrassment, tiredness, or an initial lack of motivation. This can be addressed by discussing the need for them to prioritize their sessions together in order to ensure that they occur, as therapy will not be successful without this. They should also be informed that many couples find things a little difficult initially.

Major blocks are less common but very important. The successful management of these is crucial within sex therapy, and perhaps

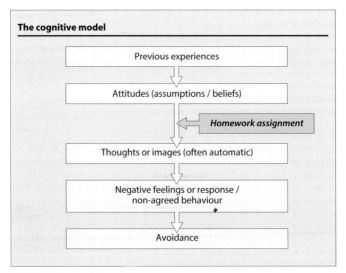

FIGURE 5. The cognitive model.

the core skill of an effective sex therapist. They should be addressed using a cognitive model, as shown in Figure 5.

The automatic negative thoughts or images which occur and cause blocks to sexual activity may concern the nature of the assignment or the possible consequences as perceived by the patient(s) concerned. The therapist should help the couple to identify automatic thoughts and images, then identifying underlying attitudes or beliefs and encouraging the partners to review evidence for them whilst considering alternative and more helpful interpretations of the situation. Myths and misunderstandings regarding sex are often exposed at this point, so that it is very important to have sessions in clinic with both partners being present if at all possible. Sometimes it may become necessary to alter the focus of therapy temporarily, in order to address the problems encountered, returning to the sensate focus approach at an appropriate later time. Table 6 may assist the therapist in trying to facilitate progress in sex therapy.

Dealing with blocks to therapy

Strategies for minor difficulties
1. Acknowledge difficulty and offer encouragement
2. Suggest easier or alternative homework assignments

Strategies for major difficulties
1. Identify negative thoughts and attitudes
2. Interpretation
3. Explore a series of explanations

Other useful strategies
1. Identify the positive benefits of homework assignments
2. Attribute positive intentions to actions
3. Positive relabelling/reframing of events[1]
4. Reassurance about normality of experiences
5. Giving permission[2]
6. Paradoxical intention[3]
7. Seeing the partners individually
8. Confrontation[4]

TABLE 6. Dealing with blocks to therapy. From Hawton, K. (1985) *Sex Therapy: A Practical Guide*. Reprinted by permission of Oxford University Press.

[1]Positive relabelling/reframing of an event means discussing an event, which is initially seen as negative by the patient, in such a way as to show the positive side of it – for example, as a useful experience or as helpful in illustrating the nature or cause of the sexual problem.

[2]Giving permission, in this context, means discussing sex, sexual activity or sexual preferences in an accepting and positive manner, effectively allowing or giving permission for the patient to also see these issues as important and acceptable.

[3]The use of paradox is a technique which was first developed in systems/family therapy work (Selvini Palazolli *et al.*, 1978). It should be used with care, in selected cases (often this means those which fail to progress with any other approach), and possibly only by a specialist in this area. In essence, it involves giving a suggestion to the couple which may appear contrary to the goal of therapy but which the therapist feels may in fact lead to progress. One simple example might be to suggest that a couple who have been striving to arouse each other should avoid arousal. Another would be to describe or summarize a particular and apparently intractable problem in the couple's relationship, but then say that it should stay as it is rather than that the couple should try to change it. This can focus the couple's efforts upon what remains, to them, a problem worth tackling.

[4]On occasion it may also be necessary to confront a lack of progress in a very direct way (e.g. if sessions are simply not occurring). The reasons behind this may be elucidated but it is also important to be clear with the couple that, analogous to taking antibiotics for a chest infection, progress will only be possible if the treatment is actually applied. Although the sex therapy approach described in this book will enable clinicians to help many patients with sexual problems, there are obviously also frequent cases which require more specialized techniques and perhaps referral on to a specialist psychosexual medicine service.

iii) Education

This will occur informally throughout clinic sessions with the couple. Sexual anatomy, physiology and response should be discussed and clarified. It may also be helpful to suggest reading for the couple, using a general text (e.g. *The Book of Love* by Delvin, 1974), or specific texts (e.g. *Men and Sex* by Zilbergeld, 1978 or *Becoming Orgasmic* by Heiman and LoPiccolo, 1999), depending upon the specific problems occurring.

A specific education session is also helpful in most cases, being tailored to the educational level, age and cultural background of the individuals concerned. This may occur a few sessions into treatment, perhaps around the time of commencing genital sensate focus. The aim of this is to provide information and dispel sexual myths (such as those listed on page 43), to alleviate anxieties and enhance understanding and confidence, and to identify any important blind spots or fallacies which might perpetuate the couple's problems. Diagrams and photographs may be a helpful adjunct.

It is important throughout therapy to be flexible regarding the approach and to adjust the pace of progress through the stages to best suit each couple and their particular difficulties. As with any psychotherapy approach it is also important to prepare for termination from the start of therapy. This can be assisted by extending the intervals between later sessions, attempting to prepare the couple for future problems which could arise and which they might now be able to deal with more effectively, and perhaps setting a follow-up assessment for some 3 months after the final treatment session.

Specific techniques for specific conditions

Many of the possible sexual dysfunctions with which a therapist might be faced can be dealt with by applying specific techniques in parallel with, or on the background of, the general sex therapy approach just described. These specific techniques will now be described in more detail, under the headings of sexual dysfunctions to which they apply, and each for problems in women and men in turn.

Lack or loss of sexual interest

IN WOMEN OR MEN

Despite the fact that the terms 'drive' and 'desire' are often used interchangeably by patients and professionals when discussing sexual feelings, they are not the same. Drive is a fundamental biological urge which is not subject-specific, whose total absence is suggestive of an organic pathology. Desire is subject-specific (i.e. usually about a specific person) and can be variable in intensity or even absent without this reflecting the presence of pathology, whether physical or psychological. Thus, it is possible to experience loss of or absence of desire without loss of drive, so that a person may lose interest in sex with their partner while continuing to have sexual thoughts and feelings from time to time. It is always important to elicit in the history and mental state examination which of these is present or altered, in order to consider physical versus psychological problems in the aetiology of a loss or lack of sexual interest. It is also important to remain alert to the tendency to categorize the partner with a lower sexual interest as having a problem, despite the fact that this will not necessarily be either helpful or accurate.

Treatment for a total *loss of drive* may be the identification and treatment of an organic disorder, such as testosterone deficiency. This treatment, or hormonal augmentation in peri- or post-menopausal women, should only be undertaken by suitably medically qualified professionals such as endocrinologists or gynaecologists.

Treatment for a *loss of desire*, in both men and women, is based on addressing the specific areas of difficulty identified in the assessment and formulation. It is important to be as clear as possible about the aetiology of the loss of desire. It is very often secondary to general relationship problems, or a consequence of the fact that the couple's lives may have changed and become much busier over the years. The result can be that they spend very little time together at all. '*Timetabling*' is a useful technique when trying to find out whether this process of 'growing apart' is the problem, and to demonstrate it to the couple. Each of them is asked to complete a timetable covering every hour of all seven days of a typical week, and to classify the time according to the following categories:

- Work at work (employment)
- Work at home (including housework, etc.)
- Family time
- Extended family time
- Social time (with friends)
- Couple time (just the two of them)
- Personal time (for the individual)

They are then (perhaps between the next two sessions) asked to do the same for a typical week at a time in the past, before their problem(s) arose. The results are often striking and quite powerful with regard to increasing understanding of the problem and motivating the couple to address it (Butcher, 1999). In fact, it should be recommended to all busy/active couples who have been together for several years. It is a very effective way of illustrating the need to remain aware of the importance of setting time aside to be together as a couple. A relationship in which couple time is virtually nil is not conducive to a healthy and satisfying sex life.

If the loss of desire is indeed a consequence of **general relationship problems**, these must be addressed in order to allow the later rebuilding of a satisfactory sexual relationship through sensate focus. Such relationship problems are approached through **couple work**, aimed at facilitating an equal discussion in which both parties can put across their point of view and be heard. Various techniques may be employed in this regard, including making lists of the aspects of the other partner's behaviour or personality that are cherished or disliked, considering priorities and whether these coincide, and timetabling (as above). Apart from identifying a basic lack of time together, the couple may discuss the fact that when they are together they are very tired. This can be a good basis upon which to discuss what sort of life together they actually want, and can realistically achieve. This is of course likely to change as their lives progress: people with small children, in jobs which do not synchronize free time, or who are caring for elderly relatives, may begin to understand more clearly why their partnership is suffering.

The roles people adopt throughout their lives may also influence how they see themselves and how their partner sees them. Taking women as the example, the range of interpersonal roles through which they pass might be listed as follows:

- Daughter
- Sister
- Friend
- Work colleague
- Girlfriend
- Lover
- Wife
- Mother
- Grandmother, etc.

Any one individual will obviously occupy several roles at any one time. The problem is that, for some people, certain roles are more immediately powerful than others, in terms of how the individual sees herself (self-identity) and the impact this has upon behaviour. In particular, the mother role may virtually eclipse all others, and particularly may be viewed as much more important than the lover role. Behaviour in and around the sexual relationship which seems acceptable as a young lover lacking many responsibilities may just not be seen as appropriate for a mother of young children. This tends, of course, to be an unconscious problem, manifesting in a loss of interest in sex, with potential wider relationship problems as a result. It may be particularly striking in a person who perceived her own mother (perhaps her only model for that role) to be serious, judgmental and sexless. Such issues will need to be addressed if they are an important part of the aetiology of a loss of interest in sex.

Often, in the case of general relationship problems, simply improving communication and allowing the two partners to express themselves freely in a non-threatening environment, with facilitation by a third party, is enough to begin a process which, if fostered, strengthens honesty, trust and respect on both sides. As communication improves the therapist may 'withdraw' more and more from the conversation (perhaps in part physically by rearranging the three chairs), in order to allow the couple to communicate directly with each other more effectively than has been possible for them for some time.

In their popular textbook, *Therapy with Couples*, Crowe and Ridley (2000) describe the overall goals of such therapy:
- Improved couple adjustment (communication, negotiation and satisfaction)
- Increased flexibility of interaction in the relationship
- Reduction of any symptoms or individual problems
- Decrease in labelling one partner as the 'problem'

- If the relationship or the individual problems cannot be improved, reduce expectations and 'live with it'
- Any improvement should be able to last without further therapeutic help

It would not be appropriate to expand upon the elements of couple therapy in this book, but for those interested in reading more, Crowe and Ridley's book is recommended (see Appendix, page 94).

Another problem which may be encountered is that of one or other partner complaining that they no longer find their partner attractive. If this is the case they will have to consider what their options are, and whether or not the relationship should continue. Before this decision is reached, and to help the person to think through this problem, it may be helpful for them to consider what brought them together originally, under the following three headings:

- Attraction
- Goals (i.e. what they want out of life, what they want to do or achieve)
- Beliefs (i.e. what life is about, what is important, how one should live and behave)

In considering these areas an individual will not uncommonly find that they do in fact want to remain with their partner, and will engage in looking at ways to address their relationship problems and to maximize the success of the physical part of their relationship. This will occur if they still see a high level of 'closeness of fit' between them and their partner, despite a perception that immediate physical attraction has diminished. On occasions, of course, the declared loss of attraction and interest may remain, and may ultimately lead to the end of the relationship.

Still regarding the problem of a lack of sexual interest, recent years have seen the emergence of a very important and helpful *alternative model of sexual response in women*. Rosemary Basson in Canada has written extensively about the need to avoid the assumption that women ordinarily engage in sexual activity simply in response to an underlying desire for sex itself. Her work has shown that women may engage in sex with a partner for a broad range of other reasons, including wanting to increase emotional closeness, commitment, sharing, tenderness and tolerance, and to show the partner that he or she has been missed, whether emotionally or physically (Basson, 2001). Such 'intimacy-based reasons', rather than actual sexual desire, motivate the woman to find a way initially to become sexually aroused with her partner. Once arousal begins, sexual desire itself may arise in the setting of ongoing sexual activity. In other words, sexual interest or desire can emerge ***during*** sex even though it was not present at all before the sex started (Figure 6). It can be helpful to explain to a couple that the woman's relative lack of sexual interest, other than during an episode of sex, may be perfectly normal, as this is the general pattern in large

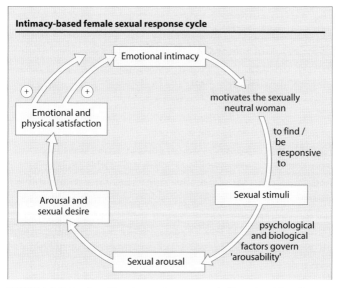

FIGURE 6. Intimacy-based female sexual response cycle. Reproduced from Basson, R. (2001) Drugs for sexual dysfunction. *Obstet Gynecol* **98**(2): 350–353 with permission from Lippincott, Williams & Wilkins.

numbers of women. This can be a particularly helpful way to conceptualize the problem in a couple, for example, who complain that he always initiates sex and she never does, so that she 'must therefore have a problem with a lack of sexual interest', or because she does not desire him between episodes of sex. In such cases, it is common for the woman to immediately recognize the 'Basson model' (as just outlined) when it is described to her or the couple in clinic. Apart from reassuring them, this may be a way of normalizing their approach. When it is explained that it may simply be 'normal' for him to be someone who desires sex between episodes and initiates it as a result of that sexual desire, and for her to be someone who is generally a responder rather than an initiator, it is not uncommon for both partners to feel that they do not need to alter things after all. Other studies support this model as they have shown that despite many women having sexual thoughts only extremely rarely, they can be entirely normal in their sexual responsiveness (Cawood and Bancroft, 1996; Laumann *et al.*, 1999).

It is also worth bearing in mind that if the presenting problem is a life-long lack of interest in sex, this may be connected with the individual having not developed as a sexual person, for a range of possible reasons. In such cases, a ***sexual growth programme*** (as described on page 57) may be helpful.

Depression affecting sexual interest

If a psychiatric contributory factor such as loss of libido as a component of a depressive illness is identified, this also needs to be treated. Ideally, this should occur using approaches which minimize the use of medication because of the risk of further suppressing sexual interest, as a side-effect of such medication. It should be remembered that if the lack of sexual desire is of great importance to the patient, an antidepressant-induced impairment of libido may mask the degree of recovery from the depressive illness. Virtually all antidepressants, and lithium, may have the effect of decreasing sexual interest. In contrast, there is some evidence to suggest that trazodone may increase libido in both men and women who are depressed, with one study reporting that it improved libido and erections in two-thirds of patients studied (Kurt *et al.*, 1994).

Drugs affecting sexual interest

Many drugs, both prescribed and illicit, can affect sexual interest. The list includes (Bazire, 2001; Taylor *et al.*, 1997; Clayton and Shen, 1998):

- Antidepressants (clomipramine and other tricyclic anti-depressants; serotonin-specific reuptake inhibitors; venlafaxine; monoamine oxidase inhibitors; etc.)
- Lithium
- Anxiolytics and hypnotics (e.g. benzodiazepines)
- Anticonvulsants
- Acamprosate
- Antipsychotics (may help to restore libido impaired by untreated schizophrenia but have a deleterious effect on erectile and orgasmic performance and satisfaction)

If sexual interest is being suppressed by a drug, this contributory factor requires careful discussion between the patient, the therapist and the prescribing doctor, in order to weigh up the pros and cons of continuing, trying an alternative or stopping the treatment. Restoring sexual interest may be important but interfering in the prescribing relationship between the patient and another doctor without full consultation is obviously not appropriate. This is also an area in which informed consent is very important.

PROGNOSIS OF IMPAIRED SEXUAL INTEREST

Of all the types of sexual dysfunction, low sexual desire has the least favourable prognosis (Bancroft, 1998). For women this condition has a particularly poor long-term outcome. Although initial resolution of the problem (at the end of therapy) has been reported as approximately 30%, at follow-up 1–6 years later, only some 3% remain free of the problem (Hawton *et al.*, 1986). This may in part be due to some affected women having psychological issues around low self-esteem, or perhaps because the loss of sexual interest is a consequence of ongoing problems in general (non-sexual) aspects of the relationship. It is important, as with all psychological management, to remember to see the patient as a whole, not view the psychosexual problem in isolation.

Impaired arousal

IN WOMEN

In pre-menopausal women, in the absence of impaired sexual interest, impaired physiological arousal (vaginal engorgement and lubrication) appears to be relatively uncommon (Gebhard, 1978). Alternatively, it may be more common as a problem than realized but not complained of, possibly in part because it is less obvious than impaired sexual arousal in men (erectile dysfunction). When assessing the problem it is important to establish at what point during sex the impaired arousal occurs.

The partner's sexual technique may be unhelpful through inhibiting arousal, or expectations on the part of either partner may be unrealistic. Discussion and challenging of the '*myths of sexuality*' may be helpful in such circumstances (Zilbergeld, 1978). Such myths are relevant with regard to **both men and women** (Table 7).

It can be useful for the woman to share with her partner her own experience of successful arousal techniques. In general, and in the absence of an organic cause for the arousal impairment (e.g. diabetes, multiple sclerosis, severe vascular disease or any of the list of medications which are known to impair arousal, as listed on page 46), the approach to this area of difficulty follows the usual sensate focus pattern, with promotion of communication about sexual matters. The sharing of responsibility for sexual arousal between the couple will also be important.

Myths of sexuality
1. Sex should be natural and spontaneous – asking for it spoils it
2. All physical contact must lead to sex
3. Men always want and are ready for sex
4. Sex is for male pleasure – a woman's duty is to fulfil his need not her own
5. Men must take charge of and orchestrate sex
6. If women aren't orgasmic they should fake it
7. Women expect men to know all about sex
8. Men should not have or at least not express certain feelings
9. Anything other than the missionary position is dirty
10. Women must wait for the male to initiate
11. For men, in sex, as elsewhere, it is performance that counts
12. Women must maintain a 'good' reputation
13. Women must be attractive, obedient and passive – because men expect it
14. Having sex means having intercourse
15. For the couple to have sex, the man must have an erection
16. Good sex always ends in orgasm
17. Good sex means both partners having an orgasm, preferably at the same time
18. There is something wrong with a man who has a lower sex drive than a woman
19. In general, women receive more stimulation from a large penis than a small one
20. Nice girls don't get turned on – and they certainly never move during lovemaking
21. Don't show affection to men because they will want sex
22. If a woman shows interest in making love, she must be promiscuous
23. Most homosexuals exclusively adopt the passive or active role in their sexual relationship
24. In this enlightened age, none of the previous myths have had any effect on any of *us*

TABLE 7. Myths of sexuality.

Where there are ongoing difficulties stemming from previous sexual traumas, individual work to help the woman deal with these may be indicated. If psychodynamic or similar techniques are required, sensate focus may have to be postponed while this individual work is carried out. In such circumstances, and as far as allowed by the woman concerned, explanation to the partner as to what the problem is and why most physical activity is being postponed can be very helpful.

There are various ways in which the woman or couple may attempt to maximize arousal. Sexual fantasies can be a mechanism to increase arousal but need a tactful and considered approach if they are to be suggested at all. Some couples may react with horror or see using fantasies as a betrayal of their partner and threat to the relationship. It can be helpful to explain in such cases that sexual arousal achieved through the use of fantasy becomes associated with the partner and their own relationship with practice, and as this association strengthens the need for the use of fantasy may reduce. Whilst always being careful to only suggest anything to a patient or couple which will not cause distress in that particular case, the therapist may consider artificial lubricants, and erotic literature, videos or vibrators as further ways to help the couple maximize sexual arousal (see Appendix, pages 94–95).

Post-menopausal women may benefit from gynaecological assessment for atrophic vaginitis, which usually responds to local application of oestrogen cream. This treatment should be supervised by a doctor (general practitioner or gynaecologist) experienced in its use, as should other hormone replacement therapy (HRT) treatments.

IN MEN (erectile dysfunction)

For prevalence figures of erectile dysfunction in various clinical settings see Table 1 on page 3. Erectile dysfunction with a clear *organic cause* is usually dealt with by the patient's general practitioner, or by a urologist or andrologist in secondary care. Ageing, vascular (arterial) disease, neurological disease, trauma, post-surgical complications and diabetes are just some of the possible physical causes of erectile dysfunction. In addition, a large number of drugs have side-effects which may include sexual dysfunction, and often erectile dysfunction specifically. These include antidepressants, anticholinergics, antihypertensives, antipsychotics, corticosteroids, diuretics, hypnotics, lithium carbonate, oestrogens and opiates, amongst others.

Table 8 lists some of the common agents implicated in erectile dysfunction, but this is not an exhaustive list. Wherever there is a reason to suspect the association of medication with sexual dysfunction, the relevant datasheets and your local Drug Information Service should be consulted for advice about alternatives as well as data about previous reports of sexual dysfunction associated with specific medication. Where necessary, a report should then be submitted to the Committee on Safety of Medicines (through the 'yellow card' system).

Impact of psychotropic medication

In psychiatric practice it is particularly important to bear in mind the impact that prescribed medication may have on the desire, arousal and orgasm of patients. All too often patients are too embarrassed to raise these issues themselves, so doctors (and other healthcare professionals) need to ensure that they ask about them in an appropriate manner, regardless of whether the patient currently has a partner or not. Compliance with treatment can be markedly affected if patients experience adverse sexual side-effects. Hyperprolactinaemia and other disturbance of the hypothalamic–pituitary–adrenal (HPA) axis caused by neuroleptics (and sometimes other drugs or causes) should be borne in mind, as should the different propensity of various agents to cause sexual difficulties. It should also of course be remembered that these difficulties will not be purely sexual but multiple, and effects may be long-term. Reproductive capability is particularly important to discuss with patients when obtaining informed consent for the use of such drugs. Some agents are more likely than others to cause erectile dysfunction.

Medication associated with erectile dysfunction

Type of drug	Examples	Alternative drugs with lower risk of erectile dysfunction
Antihypertensives	Beta-blockers (e.g. propanolol, atenolol); thiazide diuretics; hydralazine	Alpha-adrenergic blockers; ACE inhibitors; calcium channel blockers
Diuretics	Thiazide diuretics; potassium-sparing diuretics; carbonic anhydrase inhibitor	Loop diuretics
Antidepressants	Selective serotonin reuptake inhibitors; tricyclic antidepressants; MAOIs	Newer agents *may* have lower risk (e.g. nefazodone, mirtazepine) but specialist opinion may be required before changing treatment
Antipsychotics	Phenothiazines; risperidone	Newer agents *may* have lower risk (e.g. quetiapine) but specialist opinion may be required before changing treatment
Mood stabilizers	Carbamazepine; lithium	
Hormonal agents	Cyproterone acetate; luteinizing hormone-releasing hormone analogues; oestrogens	Dependent on diagnosis and options available
Lipid regulators	Gemfibrozil; clofibrate	Statins
Anticonvulsants	Phenytoin; carbamazepine	**Need specialist neurological advice**
Antiparkinsonian drugs	Levodopa	**Need specialist neurological advice**
Dyspepsia and ulcer-healing drugs	H2 antagonists	Proton pump inhibitors
Miscellaneous	Allopurinol; indomethacin; disulfiram; phenothiazine; antihistamines; phenothiazine antiemetics	Cyclizine

TABLE 8. Medication associated with erectile dysfunction. NB: This table aims to suggest alternative medication which may be less likely to cause erectile dysfunction, but all the suggested alternatives are also liable to cause erectile dysfunction to some extent, and may themselves be the primary cause in a patient presenting with organic erectile dysfunction. Adapted from Ralph, D. and McNicholas, T. (2000) UK management guidelines for erectile dysfunction. *BMJ* 321: 499–503 with permission from the BMJ Publishing Group.

Buproprion, desipramine, fluvoxamine and reboxetine are all thought less likely to cause sexual dysfunction while lithium, fluphenazine, thioridazine, tricyclic antidepressants and serotonin-specific reuptake inhibitors are all commonly associated with erectile dysfunction. Smoking and alcohol consumption are common contributory factors in the aetiology of erectile dysfunction; nicotine in cigarettes may cause spasm of the penile arteries (Virag *et al.*, 1985).

A particular problem for general practitioners and psychiatrists is young men with psychosis who, upon discovering that their sexual dysfunction is related to their antipsychotic medication, choose to discontinue it and may even disengage from services or conceal their illness to avoid further exposure to it. It is obviously important to discuss this potential issue with this group of patients in order to try to avoid difficulties arising through non-adherence to treatment. There may also be pressure from the patient's partner if they are troubled by such effects of the medication.

Commonly used physical treatments for erectile dysfunction

These include vacuum devices with constriction bands (see Appendix, page 95), intracavernosal injections or intraurethral pellets of prostaglandin, and oral therapy such as sildenafil citrate (Viagra) and, more recently, sublingual apomorphine (Uprima). New and more acceptable oral treatments for erectile dysfunction are becoming available at the time of writing.

The physiological mechanism of erection involves the relaxation of vascular smooth muscle in the walls of the trabecular spaces in the corpora cavernosa. Noradrenergic transmission controls the tonic contraction of this muscle in the non-erect penis, so that blockade of this control mechanism with alpha-blocking drugs will result in an erection. Alternatively, intracavernosal injection of an alpha-agonist, such as metaraminol, will cause the erect penis to detumesce. This is used in the treatment of drug-induced priapism (Stein, 1995). Largely based around this system, various drugs have been developed for use in the treatment of erectile dysfunction (Table 9).

At the time of writing, the oral therapies have a somewhat lower efficacy rate but a better side-effect profile than more locally administered medication, such as injections. It is important to inform patients about the potential side-effects of any suggested treatment, particularly where failure to respond to a problem could have severe consequences. One particularly important example is the urgent need to detumesce an erection lasting over 2 hours. Priapism of this duration is a surgical emergency due to the risk of cavernosal necrosis. It is also important to record that this has been discussed, and to emphasize to patients that they must not manipulate their dosage or use of therapy without medical advice. (Trazodone can, rarely, cause priapism as an unwanted side-effect and is sometimes used in cases of depression with erectile dysfunction, especially where an alternative antidepressant is needed because first line antidepressant treatment has induced this problem.)

Where appropriate, surgical intervention may be considered; either vascular or to correct a deformity or insert an implant. It must be understood, however, that insertion of rods, whether silastic or with hydraulics, requires virtual ablation of the cavernosal tissue. This is clearly an absolute last resort, because if the procedure fails (e.g. due to infection) and the rods have to be removed there is no erectile tissue with which to do further work.

Some patients self-medicate with a variety of 'alternative' medications such as ginseng or gingko biloba, and may use Chinese herbal medicines or other remedies. The potential for interactions with other medications must be remembered, so that enquiry should always be made about what non-prescribed substances patients are using (Medicines Control Agency, 2002).

Drug treatment of erectile dysfunction

Yohimbine is a presynaptic alpha-2 adrenergic receptor blocker which decreases sympathetic (adrenergic) and increases parasympathetic (cholinergic) activity and is thought to have a boosting effect on noradrenergic activity in the corpora cavernosal tissues. (NB: Yohimbine is not licensed for the treatment of erectile dysfunction but is still sometimes prescribed on a named patient basis.)

Alprostadil is *prostaglandin E1* and is the main intracavernosal injection agent used in the UK at present (although *papaverine* and *phentolamine* are still used occasionally). Alprostadil is also available in a transurethral form [as a pellet passed into the penile urethra, known as '*MUSE*' (*M*edicated *U*rethral *S*ystem for *E*rection)].

Sildenafil citrate (Viagra) is a phosphodiesterase type 5 (PDE-5) inhibitor. During sexual stimulation, nitric oxide, which is released from blood vessels, activates chemical messengers including cyclic GMP. These act as vasodilators and increase penile blood flow, filling the corpora cavernosa. Cyclic GMP in penile tissue is denatured by phosphodiesterase type 5. Sildenafil works by inhibiting this enzyme, so that vasodilatation continues and the erectile response is 'boosted'. In contrast to injections or pellets of prostaglandin E1, this means that sildenafil is an 'erection enhancer' rather than an 'erection inducer'. It has to be taken approximately 1 hour before sex is expected to occur and is then at peak level of effectiveness for approximately 4 hours. Sildenafil, in common with all PDE-5 inhibitors, is contraindicated in patients taking nitrates or in patients in whom vasodilatation or sexual activity are inadvisable. In addition, in the absence of information, manufacturers of the PDE-5 inhibitors contraindicate these drugs in hypotension, recent stroke, unstable angina and myocardial infarction (British Medical Association, 2004).

Tadalafil (Cialis) is also a PDE-5 inhibitor, but with a longer duration of action than sildenafil. It has a half-life of around 17 hours and is thought to be at peak level of effectiveness from approximately 30 minutes after being taken until up to 36 hours later. (This newer preparation has the same contraindications as sildenafil, as listed above.)

Vardenafil (Levitra) is the third generally available PDE-5 inhibitor. It is recommended to be taken 25–60 minutes before sexual activity (British Medical Association, 2004). Its half-life and absorption characteristics are similar to, and it has the same contraindications as, sildenafil (as listed above).

Sublingual apomorphine (Uprima) is a centrally acting dopaminergic agonist which has been introduced very recently for the treatment of erectile dysfunction in men. Nitric oxide (as mentioned above) is known to play an essential role in the production of erections evoked by central neurotransmitters/mediators. The latter include dopamine as well as oxytocin, excitatory amino acids and serotonergic ($5HT_{2c}$) agonists, hence the erectogenic effect of apomorphine.

TABLE 9. Drugs used in the treatment of erectile dysfunction.

Prescribing regulations for drug treatments for erectile dysfunction

In response to financial concerns for the National Health Service in the UK upon the introduction of Viagra (sildenafil citrate), the Department of Health (DoH) has laid out guidance regarding which patients can receive drug treatment on the NHS for erectile dysfunction. The guidance covers all currently licensed drugs and, as a recent addition, vacuum devices:

- Sildenafil (Viagra)
- Tadalafil (Cialis)
- Vardenafil (Levitra)
- Apomorphine (Uprima)
- Alprostadil (Caverject, Viridal, MUSE)
- Vacuum devices (added to the regulations April 2002)

As new drug treatments are licensed, the DoH adds them to the list.

A patient can be prescribed drug treatment for erectile dysfunction on the NHS by his general practitioner or hospital doctor if he has been receiving any therapy for erectile dysfunction since on or before 14 September 1998, or if he has one of the following concurrent conditions or falls into a specified patient group:

- Diabetes
- Multiple sclerosis
- Parkinson's disease
- Poliomyelitis
- Prostate cancer or prostatectomy
- Radical pelvic surgery
- Renal failure treated by dialysis or transplant
- Severe pelvic injury
- Single gene neurological disease
- Spinal cord injury or spina bifida

In such cases, prescribing can be transferred to the patient's general practitioner after titration to an effective dose. However, some NHS Trusts have chosen to allow the prescribing of drugs for erectile dysfunction either not at all or only by experts in the field. In either case, communication to the general practitioner to transfer care is all that is needed.

In contrast, patients who do not fall into these categories can be treated in one of two ways:

- They can receive private prescriptions from their general practitioner (which their GP cannot charge them for); or
- If they are suffering from 'severe distress' in relation to their erectile dysfunction they can receive NHS treatment from 'specialist services'.

Specialist services are defined as services commissioned locally by Primary Care Groups or Trusts and delivered through a service agreement. Usually these are mental health services, psychosexual services, urology services or genito-urinary services.

In the current guidelines, 'severe distress' is not defined apart from a statement that the diagnosis of it should require the following criteria:

- Significant disruption to normal social behaviour and occupational activity
- Marked effect on mood, behaviour, social and environmental awareness
- Marked effect on interpersonal relationships

Controversially, in the case of patients who receive treatment under the 'severe distress' criterion, treatment (i.e. prescriptions) must **continue** to be provided by a hospital specialist service. Such prescriptions can be provided in two ways:

- A hospital prescription that is dispensed by the hospital pharmacy; or
- An FP10(HP) prescription dispensed at a community pharmacy, which must be endorsed 'SLS'.

Problems have arisen because most hospitals, unlike primary care services, do not have an effective 'repeat prescription' system.

Erectile dysfunction is a chronic condition and patients may require years or even decades of treatment. This could lead to outpatient clinics becoming overloaded and blocked by patients returning for repeat prescriptions. Thus, there is a need to provide these repeats without the patient being seen every time they require a new supply of the medication. As a result, the prescriber may be unaware of any concurrent medication that the patient is taking, and there are some significant interactions with sildenafil (e.g. concurrent use with nitrates or nicorandil is contraindicated). A number of different approaches have been tried to overcome this difficulty, the most successful involving a 'prescription maintenance scheme' such as the one set up by the acute hospital pharmacy services in Leeds (Howard and Allwood, 2002).

The DoH has also given guidance on the frequency of dosing, recommending that one treatment per week should be adequate for most patients. This can be problematic for more sexually active patients or those going on holiday, so that some flexibility would seem reasonable.

Erectile dysfunction with a likely **psychological cause** (possibly coexisting with an organic cause) may be referred to a psychosexual service, where one exists. Alternatively, a general psychiatrist may be approached for their opinion and advice. Lack of an identifiable organic cause, sudden onset and a situational pattern all suggest that the problem is psychogenic (see Table 4, page 17). Depending on the 'psychological-mindedness' of the patient it may be possible to identify and address the causes of the erectile dysfunction through therapy without using adjunctive therapy such as drugs. This is not always possible, however, and an important part of the assessment is checking whether the patient shares the aims and philosophy of treatment of the psychosexual service they are engaging with. This may not be the case for a variety of possible reasons; cultural factors, educational level, intellectual capacity and conceptual framework may all be relevant here. There should be no bar to combination therapy – where drugs, or even other physical treatments, are used alongside psychological therapy if necessary. When setting up a psychosexual service it is important to consider how this will be achieved when needed. This may mean establishing good working relationships with allied services such as urology and diabetology, especially where local Trust prescribing practices may dictate that only certain specialties can prescribe drugs for erectile dysfunction.

Psychological approaches to the treatment of erectile dysfunction
These involve identification and resolution of marital/couple conflict and the sensate focus approach for couples, as previously described. It is also important to assess whether the problem (as is often the case in psychogenic erectile dysfunction) is one of *performance anxiety* (Figure 7).

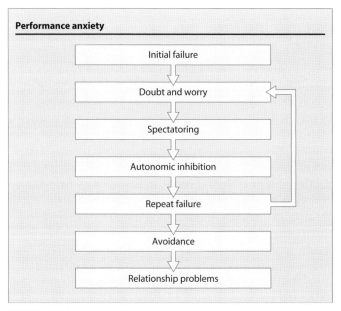

FIGURE 7. Performance anxiety.

'*Spectatoring*' refers to the process of psychologically or emotionally 'standing back' from what is happening during sex, to 'observe' (and worry about) one's own sexual 'performance' (e.g. strength of erection). In other words, the person is having anxious rather than sexually stimulating cognitions. The result is an inhibition of the usual feedback loop of sexual arousal, via interference with stimulation of the genital vasculature by autonomic nerves. The initial 'failure' of erectile functioning may have had various causes, such as anxiety, excessive alcohol, environmental factors (cold), etc., but the resultant spectatoring sets up a cycle of repeating failure, as shown in the diagram.

If performance anxiety is the problem, a description of it using the above diagram will lead to recognition and confirmation by the person concerned. Sensate focus can then be used (as described earlier) to help the couple rebuild their sexual relationship without performance anxiety causing problems.

Men who do not have a sexual partner but have a problem with erectile dysfunction may find themselves in something of a 'catch-22' situation. They may avoid or fail to secure relationships as a result of their sexual dysfunction, but have no setting within which to use sensate focus techniques to overcome it. In the past, this situation was often made worse by the fact that sex therapy was not offered to single people, only to couples. The modern day approach is to offer help with sexual problems to whoever presents to services, whether in a relationship or not. Having said that, in the case of erectile dysfunction at least, a psychological (behavioural) approach in a single man has definite limitations. What can be offered is explanation and education (the formulation) as a means of reducing anxiety, plus a simple technique to increase the man's confidence in his erectile functioning, called 'waxing and waning'. The latter involves pausing during masturbation and allowing the erection to reduce before continuing masturbation with a return of the erection. This is obviously only a useful possibility in men with situational erectile dysfunction. Doing this several times during each masturbation session can improve confidence, however, and show that the normal lessening of the strength of an erection which will occur at times during love making does not necessarily signify the impending loss of the erection altogether. In addition, of course, medication may help to reduce avoidance of future liaisons or relationships as it also can have a beneficial effect upon the patient's confidence in his ability to have an erection if the need arises.

PROGNOSIS OF IMPAIRED AROUSAL

With psychosexual treatment

Research suggests that successful resolution of the problem will occur in around 75% of those treated, with 60% remaining in remission at follow-up between 1 and 6 years later (Hawton and Catalan, 1986). This is not as high a resolution rate as in original work by Masters and Johnson. Having said that, it does represent a good rate of success, and in a population much less selected and less intensively treated than the patients in those earlier treatment studies.

With physical treatments

Intracavernosal injections may achieve beyond 90% technical success but are often unacceptable to patients (and partners), with priapism, penile pain and fibrosis as recognized complications (Ralph and McNicholas, 2000). Vacuum devices may be more acceptable, though they require some dexterity and practice to master successfully and the cost of the equipment may be off-putting for some patients. The introduction of the newer oral agents for the treatment of erectile dysfunction has widened the range of treatment options and boosted success rates for the treatment of erectile dysfunction. In patients treated with sildenafil, 50–88% of patients report improvement in erectile response, and provided the appropriate prescribing precautions are in place, sildenafil appears to be safe (Ralph and

McNicholas, 2000). At the time of writing the only newer oral agent is sublingual apomorphine, with a 67% success rate being reported from early trial work (Morales, 2001).

Surgical interventions, including implantation of silastic rods or rods with hydraulic systems, are outside the scope of this book, but it is worth noting that both technical success and patient and partner satisfaction rates are high with penile implants (Ralph and McNicholas, 2000). As mentioned earlier, however, it is essential to appreciate that such intervention involves the total ablation of cavernosal tissue, so that failure has serious implications.

Difficulties with orgasm

IN WOMEN

Range of orgasmic response

It is important to understand that there is a range of orgasmic response in women. A significant proportion of women rarely or never reach orgasm. Most surveys suggest that some 7–10% of women have never had an orgasm (Hunt, 1975; Kinsey *et al.*, 1953; Tavris and Sadd, 1977; Masters *et al.*, 1995). For some this is a problem, while for others there is no significant distress or concern. For example, one study described (in a non-random sample of couples) that 63% of women reported arousal and/or orgasm disorders – though 'happily married' – and 85% were satisfied with their sexual relationship (Frank *et al.*, 1978). Thus, orgasmic problems do not necessarily mean that sexual dissatisfaction or relationship distress will follow. Cultural factors play a large part in forming the individual woman's expectations in this area, as do her own religious and personal beliefs, values and experiences. There has been a significant and continuing increase in the level of interest displayed in this area by the media, and sometimes the resulting proliferation of articles, tapes and books about female orgasm can be helpful – but for some it causes further problems. This is particularly the case when a woman feels that she is expected to 'perform', and when partners believe that every woman should be orgasmic and judge their own sexual performance by the response of the woman concerned.

For those who are orgasmic but find their orgasmic capacity impaired, Kegel's (pelvic floor) exercises to strengthen the pubococcygeus muscle may help by improving sexual sensation and response. Where a woman is not orgasmic, thorough assessment should indicate which areas need to be addressed. For example, some women 'switch off' when highly aroused. This loss of arousal may indicate that exploration is needed to address any fear associated with orgasm, such as anxiety regarding 'losing control', so that there may be a need for individual psychological therapy. In other cases, improvements in sexual technique achieved through sensate focus exercises may be sufficient.

Some women who present with either anorgasmia or a perceived lack of sexual interest will actually give a history of very little sexual experience or none at all. There may be a sense of anxiety, fear or revulsion with regard to even the idea of engaging in sexual intercourse. This may have prevented them having any experiences with a partner, but they may now have decided that they wish to resolve this problem. In such cases a '*sexual growth programme*' can be very helpful, and often essential if any progress is to be made. (It could also be argued that most people, whether suffering a classifiable sexual dysfunction or not, might benefit from elements of such a programme.) In essence, a sexual growth programme is a way to address an individual's anxieties and psychological discomfort about sex in a graded and organized way. It has similarities to systematic desensitization and should be taken forward at a pace which is acceptable to, and largely set by, the patient herself. It must begin with education about sexual anatomy and functioning, particularly the very wide variation in the appearance of female external genitalia. This should be accompanied by discussion of fears and concerns with regard to sex, using a calm 'permission giving' approach. There will then follow a series of homework tasks, at an appropriate pace, with continuing discussion and cognitive troubleshooting of blocks in subsequent sessions with the therapist. The tasks follow a sequence:

1. **General self-examination**, possibly needing to start by spending some time **looking** at oneself in a mirror, initially clothed but later moving on to viewing oneself naked. This may be very difficult for the patient so that encouragement and working through of issues highlighted will be necessary. Later, examination of the body in general by **touching** will occur.

2. **Genital self-examination**, again initially by **looking** (e.g. with a hand mirror) and later by **touching** and digital exploration. Many women find the stages of this approach easier if they occur after relaxation, whether by specific techniques or simply a long bath.

The two examination stages are a way to help the woman become comfortable with her own body, with her genitals and with herself as a sexual being. Most women will readily agree that they need to be able to achieve this before they will be able to be comfortable with another person in a sexual situation and allow the closeness and intimacy which they may be looking for.

3. **Touching for pleasure**, with discussion of issues or problems encountered in therapy sessions.

4. **Enhancing sexual arousal**, particularly for women wishing to achieve orgasm for the first time. It is very important to be careful, tactful and aware of the patient's views as to what is acceptable before considering discussion of erotic literature or the possible use of a vibrator (see Appendix, pages 94–95).

5. **Sharing discoveries with the partner** (if there is one), and dealing again with concerns or difficulties which might arise.

Helpful reading may be suggested to the patient, such as Heiman and LoPiccolo's *Becoming Orgasmic,* which is also recommended by Relate and the Family Planning Association. This is not a short self-help manual but many women find the stages of a sexual growth programme as outlined in that particular text to be both accessible and helpful (Heiman and LoPiccolo, 1999; see Appendix, page 94).

Prognosis of female anorgasmia

Few figures are available as to outcome with therapy. One study reports a good level of response in the 'problem resolved although difficulties still experienced' category, but with very small numbers (Hawton *et al.*, 1986). Conclusions cannot really be drawn based upon the figures available. Adequate trials of treatment are still awaited (Crowe and Jones, 1992).

IN MEN

Broadly speaking, men may have five types of problem with the orgasm stage of sexual response:
1. Premature ejaculation
2. Retarded ejaculation (but able to ejaculate sometimes)
3. Retrograde ejaculation (into the urinary bladder)
4. Absent ejaculation (never ejaculates)
5. Ejaculation but with reduced or lack of central sense of orgasm

Premature ejaculation (PE)

What constitutes premature ejaculation? This is a complex question, especially because what is felt to be fine for one couple may be seen as premature by another. Perhaps the best definition would be something like 'ejaculation which occurs too soon in the subjective view of the couple concerned'. This very broad approach to conceptualizing premature ejaculation must be balanced, however, by realism. Most people would agree that ejaculation occurring before penetration or within one or two minutes thereafter would be premature. Having said that, if a man or couple present complaining that ejaculation is too soon because it occurs 10 or 15 minutes after thrusting commences, the first action to take would be to educate and facilitate discussion around realistic expectations. Those writing in the American literature are beginning to use the term 'rapid ejaculation' as an alternative.

Premature ejaculation is usually best treated with a behavioural approach such as that used in the excellent self-help manual *How to Overcome PE* by Helen Singer Kaplan (Kaplan, 1989; see Appendix, page 94). This incorporates 'masturbation training' and the 'stop–start technique' (otherwise eponymously described as Seman's technique). The theoretical basis for this approach is that the fundamental problem in premature ejaculation is an ***inability to control the ejaculatory reflex***. The key to success in treatment is for the man to become proficient in identifying the 'moment of ejaculatory inevitability' (i.e. the point at which the man can sense that ejaculation is imminent and when even a cessation of all sexual activity would fail to prevent it). The patient is likely to readily understand this as 'the point of no return'.

Many patients suffering with premature ejaculation will already have tried distraction techniques during sex as a way to try to delay ejaculation. Typically these include such things as thinking non-sexual thoughts (e.g. about cricket or a problem at work) or inflicting pain on oneself by pinching. Other common techniques include masturbating before sex or taking a cold shower. Such attempts do not work (quite apart from the fact that they obviously reduce the man's enjoyment in sex). What is actually required is for the man to learn or train himself to control the ejaculatory reflex. This necessitates proficiency at identifying the moment of ejaculatory inevitability (MOEI), which in turn requires the man to focus upon physical genital sensations during sex. Thus, the therapist will ask him to carry out sessions of masturbation, alone and when not expecting to be disturbed. During these he will concentrate upon the pleasurable sensations in his genital area and will try to identify the MOEI. He will attempt to *stop* just before he reaches that point, and will then wait for several seconds to allow the feeling of being close to ejaculation to subside. He should not wait so long as to allow the erection to subside, and should *start* masturbation again when he no longer feels that ejaculation is very close. In this way, he should practise 'stop–start' three times, allowing himself to continue on to ejaculation the fourth time it approaches.

Going too far (failing to stop before ejaculation) should not be seen as a failure, but as a way for him to learn to accurately identify the MOEI and to improve his ability to stop just before it on the next occasion. Sessions should occur two or three times each week, with an attempt, as time goes on, to increase the duration of each session (from commencement to ejaculation), and so to begin to experience improved control. Meanwhile, if he is in a sexual relationship, the couple should continue to have physical pleasurable time together, but along non-genital sensate focus lines as described above.

When the patient has achieved improved control so that masturbation sessions can last several (e.g. 7–10) minutes, he should be instructed to continue but with a lotion on his hand during masturbation (e.g. 'baby oil' as a cheaper alternative to a vaginal lubricant). He will be likely to find that ejaculation is a little quicker under such circumstances, but should continue stop–start sessions until a reasonable degree of control is again achieved.

Stop–start can next be brought into sessions with his partner, in the setting of genital sensate focus with manual stimulation by the partner (whom he can tell or signal to in some way when a stop/pause is necessary). Later, stop–start stages are stimulation by the partner with a lotion, vaginal containment without movement (female superior position being used initially as ejaculation is generally quicker in a traditional 'missionary' position, due to the pulling down of skin at the base of the penis), and finally penetrative intercourse, but still with appropriate stop–start elements. The ultimate aim is for the man to be able to have some control over his ejaculatory reflex even by simply 'slowing down' when necessary rather than actually stopping as such.

Sometimes the patient may be unable to follow this approach. As it is generally seen as the best approach available, every effort should be made to facilitate it by additional explanation and exploration of concerns or, if there is a language difficulty, by providing translated written material. It may be that the patient simply refuses to try such an approach, sometimes despite fully understanding the rationale for it. It is pointless to try to 'force' a person to follow this approach if they have a different goal or agenda, such as taking medication to 'slow things down'. When the man is completely focused on medication or medical intervention as the solution, physical treatments can be provided (preferably as an adjunct to the behavioural approach outlined but sometimes as the sole treatment). Topical anaesthetic or 'freeze' sprays and gels have been suggested as useful and can be bought over the counter. They are not to be recommended, however, in view of their anaesthetic effects upon the vulval and vaginal tissue (or other areas) of the partner's body. A much better and often effective alternative is treatment with a serotonin-specific reuptake inhibitor (SSRI). Of these, paroxetine would seem to have most research evidence to support its use in premature ejaculation (Waldinger *et al.*, 1994; Ludovico *et al.*, 1996). This medication should be initially taken daily for 3 months and then, if effective, on an 'as required basis' on the day of sex. It must be explained to the patient, however, that this is a temporary solution in that the problem is likely to return when medication is stopped. Monitoring of side-effects is obviously important when using SSRIs in this way.

An addition to stop–start is the 'squeeze technique', as pioneered by Masters and Johnson (Masters and Johnson, 1970). Despite what many people may think, this is not a simple technique to apply correctly. It is very anatomically specific and if incorrectly used (which is easy to do) it can cause discomfort and can therefore be ineffective. Thus, given that stop–start is very often successful without it, it may be best in general to avoid using the squeeze technique.

Prognosis of premature ejaculation Premature ejaculation has the best prognosis of any condition treated with sex therapy. With the behavioural treatments, a 96% success rate is reported by Hawton *et al.* (1986), while Kaplan claims that "over 90% of premature ejaculators can be cured within an average of 14 weeks of treatment". This 'cure rate' refers to initial remission, however, so that the patient's new learnt skills may be needed again in the future if there is a problem with relapse.

Retarded ejaculation

Conventionally, retarded ejaculation has been considered to be a consequence of the man 'holding back' or at least being unable, for psychological reasons, to ejaculate in the presence of a woman or intravaginally. This may be due to a specific problem between the couple concerned, or because of a more general problem on the part of the male partner himself. Some men may develop a strikingly dichotomized view of women. In other words, they may view all women as belonging to one of two 'groups' or 'types'. These are (a): 'easy', dirty, bad, sexually available women (akin to a very traditional view of a 'whore') and, in contrast, (b): good, clean, virtuous, mother-like women. They may see it as reasonable to have sex with, and ejaculate in the presence of, type (a) but certainly not type (b). Considering the fact that they may tend to choose a woman of the second type as their wife/life-partner/mother for their children, it is perhaps unsurprising that a problem with ejaculation and sex may arise in that relationship. Other psychological formulations have been advanced for failure to ejaculate. Psychoanalytically, it is felt to be an expression of the patient's unconscious fears of the dangers associated with ejaculation, while systems theory suggests that the key lies in understanding the meaning of the symptom in terms of the effect on the relationship between the sexual partners.

More recently these traditional views of psychogenic retarded ejaculation have been challenged, partly in response to difficulties treating it successfully with the types of conceptualization just outlined. Apfelbaum has suggested that the problem be reformulated in a way which is based upon the concept of 'autosexuality'. That is, the idea that men with retarded ejaculation may be achieving an erection satisfactory for intercourse automatically in response to a certain situation, without actual subjective sexual arousal. Because many men who experience retarded ejaculation with their partner can achieve orgasm when they are alone, the problem of retarded ejaculation might be viewed as 'partner anorgasmia' [i.e. situational anorgasmia with a partner (Apfelbaum, 2000)]. The suggestion is that retarded ejaculation has been inappropriately treated by viewing it as almost analogous to vaginismus in women, using a behavioural approach which produces a tremendous pressure to perform to orgasm amounting almost to 'sexual coercion'. It may be preferable to view it like female anorgasmia, in which the focus is on the negative emotions of the woman towards her partner, her fears and underlying feelings. Apfelbaum suggests that the way forward is to openly help the man to face his negative feelings rather than go on denying them (i.e. hostility towards or distance from the partner and consequent lack of arousal), along with the introduction and maximization of sexual arousal itself.

In the case of retarded ejaculation presenting as an infertility problem, this is sometimes treated with superstimulation as described by Masters and Johnson, or a high speed vibrator applied to the glans penis (Crowe, 1998). Desipramine, neostigmine and yohimbine have all been suggested to be of benefit. When none of the above have worked, digital prostate massage may be suggested. If unacceptable or unsuccessful this may sometimes lead to a urologist undertaking electro-ejaculatory stimulation. Rectal vibratory excitation (with great caution to avoid damage) might also be considered.

Prognosis of retarded ejaculation Retarded ejaculation is often difficult to treat, either for psychological reasons as outlined above or because it is a side-effect of medication (i.e. those medications which reduce sexual interest or arousal, as listed on page 46). Its prognosis when treated with sex therapy is also somewhat unclear due to a lack of published data. What figures are available suggest a possible resolution rate of around 50%, but these are based on very small numbers (Hawton and Catalan, 1986). Prognosis also appears to be related to severity, to whether the condition is primary or secondary and to the existence of concomitant marital/relationship discord.

Retrograde ejaculation

Retrograde ejaculation occurs when there is a failure of the bladder neck sphincter to close at the start of ejaculation. Seminal fluid will thus pass up into the bladder instead of being emitted from the external urethral meatus, so that the patient may complain of a 'dry run'. If suspected, this problem can be confirmed by the presence of sperm in the urine. It may be helpful to ask the patient whether his urine is cloudy after sex, or to arrange for a sample to be examined under a microscope. Retrograde ejaculation may be caused by surgery to the bladder neck, prostatectomy, division or impairment of the sympathetic nerve supply, or blockade of the alpha-1 drive to the bladder neck (by medication). Diabetic neuropathy and the side-effects of some antipsychotic medication are particularly important causes to consider. Retrograde ejaculation has been reported with chlordiazepoxide, various neuroleptics (including chlorpromazine, fluphenazine, perphenazine, pimozide, thioridazine, clozapine and trifuoperazine), monoamine oxidase inhibitors, tricyclic antidepressants, trazodone, and narcotics (Hutchison *et al.*, 2002). It is possible to retrieve sperm from the bladder and wash it (through a specialized process) if fertility is an issue.

Absent ejaculation

Absent ejaculation (i.e. never occurring at all despite high arousal) should lead to physical examination and investigation, as it may indicate a physical (possibly neurological) disorder.

Lack or loss of central sense of orgasm

Some male patients, albeit rarely, present complaining that although ejaculation/emission does occur they do not, or no longer, experience a subjective 'central' sense of orgasm or climax. The most appropriate approach in such a case would be broad and pragmatic, ruling out any organic (again possibly neurological) cause, before thoroughly assessing the person with regard to issues of sub-maximal arousal, relationship problems or depression.

Sexual pain or 'dyspareunia'

IN WOMEN

This symptom always indicates the need for full assessment to exclude an organic cause and it may be necessary for this to be carried out by a gynaecologist. A careful history is essential, paying particular attention to the location of the pain (superficial/external or deep/internal) and when it began. Those carrying out a vaginal examination, or any other intimate examination, must remain cognizant of the need to have an appropriate chaperone present throughout.

Possible physical causes of superficial/external dyspareunia include infective problems, such as candida (thrush) or herpes virus type I or II, and it is also thought that subclinical human papilloma virus (wart virus) may cause an inflammatory reaction in the vagina and vulval skin, causing a burning sensation during penetrative sex. Generalized skin disorders such as eczema and psoriasis may also cause inflammatory skin reactions in the vulval area, causing soreness. Another possibility to consider is vestibulitis, characterized by specific tenderness over the tiny vestibular glands inside the vaginal entrance posteriorly. Scarring of the perineum due to tearing or episiotomy in childbirth may also cause superficial/external dyspareunia. This may resolve spontaneously or be helped by steroid cream applied to the scar to aid thinning and stretching. Occasionally, however, surgical revision may be required. Allergy to any substance coming into contact with the vulva, such as bath products, spermicide, latex condoms or even the partner's semen, may cause soreness. For the older woman, postmenopausal atrophic change or the skin disorder of lichen sclerosis are additional possibilities. Urinary tract problems can also cause dyspareunia, with interstitial cystitis being an increasingly important cause.

Deep/internal dyspareunia also requires a careful history as part of the medical assessment. Associated symptoms, such as abnormal vaginal bleeding, discharge or pain at times other than during sex, increase the likelihood of a physical aetiology. Acute onset in a woman of reproductive age should alert the doctor to the possibility of an ectopic pregnancy. Other causes may be infective, such as chlamydial infection of the cervix, or acute pelvic inflammatory disease. Other pelvic pathology, including endometriosis, ovarian cysts, chronic adhesions or bowel pathology, may also cause deep dyspareunia (Balls, 2003).

Aetiology is often mixed, perhaps because pain is a symptom often associated with fear. This may be fear of the cause, fear of being damaged or simply fear of pain recurring the next time sex occurs. This is often the mechanism through which an otherwise transient physical problem (e.g. thrush) develops into a long-standing psychological one. This illustrates the importance of taking time to listen to the woman's story, so that both the physical and psychological/emotional aspects can be identified, understood and addressed. When it cannot be fully resolved by gynaecological intervention, whether medical or surgical, dyspareunia should lead to the suggestion to the woman of appropriate sexual positions which allow her greater control over the depth of penetration, such as entry from behind whilst lying on the side, or female superior.

If predominantly psychological causes are likely, after all other causes have been excluded, it is important to remember that impaired sexual arousal itself may result in painful penetration due to inadequate lubrication. This may improve as lubrication increases during intercourse, but may otherwise benefit from additional (artificial) lubrication, an ever increasing and improving range of which is available commercially. It is, however, very important to try to understand and assist with psychological problems which may be behind the impaired arousal, in addition to suggesting symptomatic approaches such as lubrication. Sometimes impaired arousal, whatever the cause, may also lead to deep pain due to repeated buffeting of the cervix (as the upper vagina has not expanded, lifting the cervix out of reach).

By far the most common psychological cause of superficial or external dyspareunia in women is 'vaginismus', as outlined in the next section.

IN MEN

Ejaculatory pain and dyspareunia are uncommon in men and require appropriate urological assessment to exclude an organic cause such as infection of the glans (balanitis), urethra, seminal vesicles, prostate or bladder. Hyperaesthesia or over-sensitivity of the glans after ejaculation is not uncommon in normal men, but the complaint of pain during intercourse suggests a physical cause which must be investigated. In common with women, men may present complaining of a lack of interest in sex which transpires to be secondary to repeated experiences of pain or discomfort (i.e. male dyspareunia). After the cause has been identified and treated, some reassurance may be necessary but otherwise recovery with regard to sexual functioning is likely to be good.

Vaginismus

The term 'vaginismus' refers to the problem of difficulty with penetrative sex as a result of involuntary spasm of the pubococcygeus muscles (surrounding the entrance to the vagina) when penetration is attempted. This occurs as a reflex reaction, due to the 'expectation' that penetration will be painful. The original aetiology may be around aversive sexual experiences, such as rape or abuse, but is often rather simpler than that. Any cause of superficial vaginal/vulval pain during intercourse can lead to the expectation that future penetration will hurt. Such causes include sex in the presence of a vaginal thrush (candida) infection, a first or early sexual experience which was painful due to a tightly closed introitus as a result of anxiety, fear of the unknown, having been 'taught' (e.g. by the mother) that sex will hurt, or simply due to clumsiness, or a poorly performed clinical vaginal examination. The involuntary muscle spasm which follows (when penetration is expected and generally with a phobic element) can be painful in itself, but clearly exacerbated by continued attempts at penetration when the vaginal introitus is, in effect, 'closed'. When presented with such problems in clinic, an additional issue to deal with is that the woman concerned may be angry or frustrated by having seen a series of physical medical specialists for multiple investigations without a diagnosis in physical terms.

There are several components to effective treatment for this condition:
- Explanation
- Addressing couple factors
- Relaxation
- Reassurance
- Desensitization

- Not forgetting psychotherapy for unresolved traumatic experiences when necessary

Early and clear explanation in the form of a formulation discussed with the patient and, whenever possible, her partner, is an essential first step. Concerns which the partner may have regarding sex should also be addressed (as he may be quite happy to be in a relationship in which penetrative sex is not possible, so that there would clearly be consequences of a resolution of the vaginismus). What then follows is basically a systematic desensitization approach, making sure that the therapist is flexible in setting up the programme and that it proceeds, at all times, at a pace set by the female patient. This sense of control and safety within the treatment programme leads to confidence which will be essential to allow successful treatment.

Desensitization may need to begin in the form of a sexual growth programme (as described on page 57). Thereafter, using learning theory as part of the explanation of the treatment, the female patient will be given homework tasks to carry out, whilst the couple agree to refrain from attempts at penetrative sex and are invited to engage in non-genital sensate focus sessions together, if acceptable to them (page 27). The homework tasks will take the patient through stages designed to help her discover that insertion of an appropriate object into the vagina can occur without continued discomfort or any adverse consequences. It is important to start small and gradually build up. The patient should never move on to a later stage until the current stage has become comfortable and problem-free. She may begin by attempting, when alone and not in a sexual way as such, to try to insert one finger. She should use lubrication (e.g. 'sensilube' or 'liquid silk' or another similar proprietory substance). She should proceed slowly, and if possible should keep her finger inserted for a few minutes – i.e. enough time to allow the anxiety experienced to subside, or at least begin to do so, in order that the next session will be easier, and so on. Kegel's exercises are a helpful adjunct (i.e.

improving tone, power and control of the pelvic floor muscles, by identification and then sessions of repeated contraction and relaxation of these muscles, gradually building up the frequency and duration of these exercises over several weeks). These help to improve the condition and awareness of activity of the muscles around the vaginal introitus, whilst also enabling the patient to recognize the difference between the sensations of vaginal muscle contraction and relaxation. It can also help, if she is having difficulty inserting her finger, for the patient to tightly contract the pelvic floor muscles with her finger at/on the introitus, as it may slip in more easily when she then relaxes.

The next stage may be to insert two fingers, or possibly a tampon. Most therapists find graded 'vaginal trainers' very useful (see Appendix, page 94). These are plastic torpedo-shaped objects in four sizes (from finger-sized to a size approximating an erect penis) so that the patient can work slowly up through the sizes. They are *not* vaginal dilators. It is crucial for the patient to understand that the model is one of learning, not dilating or stretching – as the size of the vagina is generally not the problem. The aim is, in effect, to eventually use the partner's erect penis as the final stage, but in a way which keeps the woman in control (i.e. female superior and at her pace).

It is important for therapists to identify and address blocks which may arise during treatment. Sometimes, this can occur at an early stage, when many women find initiating the introduction of their own fingers or vaginal trainers difficult. Extra encouragement, explanation and advice may suffice. Some therapists, however, may use more direct intervention: performing a therapeutic vaginal examination – during which important issues are sometimes disclosed by the patient. Alternatively, this may simply allow progress with insertion of a finger by the patient, with help and reassurance by the therapist. The involvement of a chaperone is very important, and this approach should only be carried out by suitably qualified therapists.

When treating women for vaginismus it is also important to remember that the couple's relationship may be built around the impossibility of sex and the expectation of non-consummation, which may continue to suit one or both partners. Progress with treatment of the vaginismus may, as a result, lead on to secondary sexual dysfunction in the male partner (e.g. erectile dysfunction or premature ejaculation) which may also require treatment.

Two final points of note:

1. On occasions, a general practitioner or gynaecologist may see a female patient who presents with primary vaginismus which is due to a thought or belief that her vagina is simply too small to allow insertion of anything, including an erect penis, but which responds very well to a therapeutic vaginal examination. This involves an examination being carried out carefully and sensitively whilst talking with the patient about her fears regarding the perceived vaginal abnormality. Successful internal examination with explanation and confirmation of normality may sometimes lead to a rapid improvement or resolution of the vaginismic problem.

2. In contrast, a gynaecologist may occasionally see a woman who is referred with 'intractable vaginismus' and who they need to examine under general anaesthesia. The problem may be found, after all, to be anatomical, as in the case of a particularly firm hymen which requires stretching to resolve the problem, and which will otherwise not allow insertion of a vaginal trainer. It must be stressed, however, that this is a rare occurrence (Drife, 2003).

PROGNOSIS OF VAGINISMUS

Vaginismus generally has a good outcome from treatment but the course of therapy is often far from straightforward. This is contrary to the early reports of Masters and Johnson and some successors, who reported close to 100% success – this was probably due to case selection and the intensive nature of the treatment they were able to carry out. Even in more 'real life' settings, however, outcome of sex therapy for vaginismus continues to be reported as very good, one study reporting that it is resolved or largely resolved in 79% of cases receiving sex therapy (Hawton, 1982).

Sexual aversion/phobias

Sexual aversion/phobias *per se*, in men or women, rarely present to clinics, but may be components of other sexual dysfunctions. When addressing these it is therefore important to identify and then address any phobic elements. Sometimes the phobia is related to earlier traumatic sexual experiences and this may indicate the need for specific work to deal with issues such as incest or rape. However, if the phobia is relatively straightforward, simple behavioural or cognitive behavioural techniques using imaginal and *in vivo* exposure may be a reasonable approach to take. Key to success in helping people with sexual aversion/phobia is a thorough assessment to clearly identify what element(s) of sex cause this response. This can then allow a focus upon these specific areas and issues. Unless sexual aversion is absolute, sensate focus (if well set-up and proceeded with gradually) may be a very useful approach to allow clarification of the precise problem.

Substance-induced sexual dysfunction

Substance-induced sexual dysfunction, as mentioned above, can involve both prescribed or non-prescribed (legal or illicit) drugs. Treatment involves identifying this problem and then reconsidering with the patient, and any prescribing doctor also involved, the indications or reasons for using the drug, the relationship (if any) between dose and effects, the acceptability to the patient of this and consideration of any possible alternatives to the present treatment. Alcohol, tobacco and recreational drug use are frequently implicated in sexual dysfunction but often neglected both by patients as well as enquiring professionals when considering aetiology.

Sexual dysfunction due to a general medical condition

Where sexual dysfunction is due to a general medical condition, treatment involves education and explanation to help the patient and their partner come to terms with the diagnosis. Efforts should also be made to minimize the impact of the disease on sexual functioning. Treatment for the disease may involve the use of agents which themselves contribute to sexual dysfunction, so that the patient needs to be as fully informed as possible to make the choices necessary in deciding their treatment path. Adjunctive biological therapies may be used to try to improve any sexual dysfunction. For example, many urology departments have subsidiary erectile dysfunction services to which patients with conditions such as prostate cancer can be referred to access appropriate biological therapies.

The potential impact on sexual functioning of any medical procedure or intervention should also be borne in mind. Even simple procedures such as having a cervical smear or colposcopy can produce effects in patients which healthcare professionals, whose perception of the procedure may be very different to that of the patient and their partner, may overlook or fail to recognize.

Overall prognosis in sex therapy

In general, the prognosis for sex therapy is variable between problems (as detailed for each condition, above) and between patients with the same problem, as well as between follow-up studies. Overall, approximately 50–70% of couples report substantial benefits (Bancroft, 1998). Hawton's group completed a prospective study of prognostic factors in sex therapy, finding that the **motivation for treatment** (especially in the male partner), the **quality of the non-sexual relationship** and **progress by the third therapy session** all had prognostic significance (Hawton and Catalan, 1986).

The same authors also assessed long-term outcome for sex therapy and concluded that this was excellent for vaginismus and good for erectile dysfunction, but often poor for premature ejaculation (although this can be addressed with a return to the behavioural treatment used as described previously, as each 'course' brings with it a very good initial prognosis). They also found prognosis to be especially poor for female impaired sexual interest, citing the fact that this is often secondary to general relationship problems (Hawton *et al.*, 1986). Perhaps the prognosis in such cases is, therefore, actually dependent upon identifying and effectively addressing the general relationship problems themselves (as described on page 36).

Rating scales used in psychosexual medicine

There is a general lack of use of assessment and outcome scales in this field, as shown by a recent national survey (Holland, 2002). Regarding the use of rating scales in research, however, the following are examples of scales which are useful and/or used particularly frequently:

Golombok Rust Inventory of Marital Satisfaction (GRIMS)

A 28-item self-report measure of satisfaction with the general (non-sexual) part of the relationship and functioning in that area. Despite its name, it can be used in non-married people who are in a current relationship. It is often used when considering possible aetiological factors in cases of sexual dysfunction, i.e. to be able to say whether or not they might be secondary to a generalized relationship problem (Rust et al., 1988).

International Index of Erectile Function (IIEF)

A 15-item self-report measure of erectile functioning (frequency, quality, duration, etc.), ejaculatory functioning, satisfaction and enjoyment, desire and sexual confidence. It was produced by an international consensus group and has been used very widely, particularly in research into the effects of biological treatments for erectile dysfunction. Sensitivity and specificity properties enable it to detect treatment-related changes in patients with erectile dysfunction. Found to be 'cross-culturally valid and psychometrically sound'. Linguistically validated in 10 languages (Rosen et al., 1997).

Female Sexual Functioning Questionnaire (SFQ)

A 34-item self-report measure of sexual functioning and sexual satisfaction in women. It addresses all aspects of the sexual response cycle (desire, arousal and orgasm) as well as pain, in keeping with DSM-IV diagnostic criteria (Heiman *et al.*, 2002; Pfizer Global Research and Development, 1997). Importantly, and somewhat unusually, the arousal questions generate two separate domains of 'arousal: sensation' and 'arousal: lubrication'. Both the physical and cognitive aspects of sexual response are evaluated within the questionnaire. Use of the SFQ in clinical trials in a large sample of women (some 900 in total) has demonstrated excellent psychometric properties, including discriminative and construct validity, test–retest reliability, internal consistency and sensitivity to change (Heiman *et al.*, 2002). The seven domains were identified through factor analysis and are 'desire', 'arousal: sensation', 'arousal: lubrication', 'orgasm', 'pain', 'enjoyment' and 'partner'. It is possible to analyse results at item, domain and total score level (Heiman *et al.*, 2002; Basson *et al.*, 2000).

Ethical considerations

Sexuality is a fundamentally important area in most peoples' lives. This includes you, your partner, your patient and their partner, your colleagues and so on. Increasing awareness of sexual issues (and particularly the associated human rights) means that this area is also important to your organization, at many levels from the individual care of patients in hospital to the prescription of medications which may alter fertility or sexual functioning, as well as to your individual practice and conduct as a clinician.

Sexuality can be a difficult area to approach, for many reasons. Some are to do with our own attitudes as people and professionals, and some are to do with the patient. Personal sensibilities can be affected by religious, moral and cultural values and beliefs. Some are virtually universal, such as the taboo on intercourse with pre-pubescent children, and some not, such as the acceptability of pre-marital sex, contraceptive practices, termination of pregnancy, and whether sex should actually be enjoyed for any purpose other than procreation. However, it behoves all clinicians to set aside time to consider their own personal and professional attitudes, responsibilities and prejudices, in order to try to cultivate a sensitive approach to sexual issues. Practising asking patients about these important areas not only immediately improves our overall management of patients and their partners/families, but reduces the embarrassment felt by the enquiring practitioner.

Potential areas of difficulty

It is important that doctors or anyone else working with people with sexual problems should be non-judgemental, accepting of the lifestyle choices made by their patient and their patient's partner(s), and respectful of the importance of sexuality to these people. Therapists must not impose their own principles or preferences upon patients, nor should they assume that their patient's view of what is right, wrong, good or bad in sex is necessarily similar to their own. Having said that, it is important to acknowledge that any clinician may find it difficult to work with a patient or client whose sexual preferences or practices are too alien or even disturbing to that individual clinician. One useful way to think about these concerns is to consider the difference between '*benign variation*' and '*malignant variation*' (Gordon, 1994). Although an individual may enjoy a type of sexual activity which some others would not wish to engage in, it may be viewed as an example of benign variation if many people in society would see it as acceptable. Possible examples are oral sex and anal intercourse, or perhaps 'virtually any sexual activity which occurs in private and between consenting adults'. There are other examples which would, however, be seen by the vast majority of society as wholly unacceptable under any circumstances. These would include paedophilia, and can be considered examples of malignant variation. It is important for any individual working with people with sexual problems to consider for him or herself what behaviours or preferences would fall into each of these categories. Discussion in supervision or with another colleague working in the same field can facilitate thorough consideration of the issues and the ethical dilemmas faced when there is some such aspect to the case which the clinician finds troubling. A particularly important example might be how to proceed when asked for help with an erectile dysfunction by a man with a previous conviction for sexual assault or rape.

Appropriate behaviour for clinicians

The general behaviour of any professional working in this field is also very important. He or she must behave in an appropriate way at all times: using language appropriate to the sensibilities of the patient, using a chaperone where necessary, responding as far as possible to a patient's request for therapy by a person of a particular gender. Appropriate dress, conduct and the maintenance of clear boundaries are all essential elements of good professional conduct.

Supervision and good quality record keeping are also essential, particularly when dealing with potentially sensitive subjects such as sexual dysfunction. Keeping the patient's records separate from general medical notes may help to facilitate openness on the part of the patient. In the service run by the author, patients are reassured that their notes are kept separately in the department with only a brief entry in the main hospital notes indicating that the patient has been seen in the psychosexual medicine service.

The importance of consulting the partner (whenever possible)

An important word of warning is to remember that your patient is not usually isolated and alone, so changing their sexual function is likely to impact upon their partner. It is vital to try to engage the couple wherever possible to address problems, not just for the obvious reasons of increasing the likelihood of accurate formulation and successful treatment, but to ensure that any improvement in sexual functioning will be welcomed, and understood, and will not compromise the overall relationship.

Services for sexual dysfunction

Demand for services

Attitudes towards sexuality are changing throughout society. In particular, we are seeing an increasing proportion of older adults presenting with sexual dysfunction. The recent advent of effective and relatively side-effect-free oral therapies for erectile dysfunction, as highlighted in the media, may be partly responsible for this. In addition, there is an increasing acceptance that older people need not give up the pleasures of life just because they are ageing. This is also the case for people with disabilities and from cultural groups who may have previously found it particularly difficult to present for help with sexual problems (such as Muslim Asian women whose only apparent route towards help may be via a white male general practitioner). It is also notable that different cultural groups may present in different ways with the same condition. For example, white couples in this country with the problem of non-consummation due to primary vaginismus may present in their late 30s due to a wish to have children, whereas Asian couples describe more family pressure and concern leading to a much earlier referral via infertility services.

Provision of services

Psychosexual medicine is a developing sub-specialty area. Its boundaries overlap with several other medical and surgical specialties and many of the cases seen have mixed physical and psychological aetiology. These features are shared with the sub-specialty of liaison psychiatry, as is the likelihood that demand for services will continue to grow. In the future, other branches of medicine may look to psychiatrists to develop such services. This will of course have resource implications, but should be considered and, where possible, planned for.

Some established services do exist in the public, private and voluntary sectors. A range of staff, skill mixes and specialties may be involved, including nurses, psychologists and medically qualified practitioners from psychiatry, urology, GU medicine, gynaecology, etc. Any service will be shaped by what staff are available, their degree of training for such work and their need for further training (with attendant cost implications). It is important to give some thought to facilities, including consideration of clinic hours and accessibility, privacy and soundproofing, access to good quality supervision for all staff, clerical support and all the other usual features of providing a psychological therapy service to patients.

If there is no realistic prospect of providing a dedicated psychosexual service, patients' needs in this area still need to be considered and met as far as possible. Every clinician should be alert to the sexual aspects of their patients' lives and should incorporate enquiry about this into routine assessment. As stated earlier, they should be able to make an assessment and attempt a formulation of their patient's sexual difficulties, paying attention to both organic and psychological aspects of aetiology. In what appears to be relatively straightforward cases, sensate focus and other techniques or relevant physical treatments should be used, with referral on to specific services for difficult or complex cases, or any cases where the clinician feels that he or she lacks the skills necessary to help the patient effectively.

Paraphilias

The term paraphilia refers to a sexual activity or behaviour which is statistically abnormal. For their classification, see Table 10. As attitudes towards sexual behaviour are emotionally charged in society, deviations from the norm are regarded in a pejorative way with an accompanying marked social stigma (Sims, 1988). Doctors, perhaps mainly psychiatrists, may for a variety of reasons come into contact with people exhibiting such behaviours. They may be referred for assessment or treatment, either because their sexual behaviour brings them into contact with the criminal justice system or as a result of psychological problems suffered as a result of their paraphilic tendencies. Such individuals may have strong negative feelings about themselves (e.g. guilt, shame or disgust), or significant problems with loving/long-term relationships as a result of their sexual preferences. Although this book is focused almost entirely upon sexual dysfunction, it will be worthwhile to outline details of some of the most prevalent paraphilias here.

Classification of paraphilias
Fetishism
Exhibitionism
Paedophilia *Specifiers:* • Sexually attracted to males/females/both • Limited to incest • Exclusive type/non-exclusive type
Sexual masochism
Sexual sadism
Transvestic fetishism
Voyeurism
Paraphilia NOS (not otherwise specified)
Frotteurism

TABLE 10. Classification of paraphilias. Reprinted with permission from the *Diagnostic and Statistical Manual of Mental Disorders*, fourth edition. Copyright © 2000. American Psychiatric Association.

Types of paraphilia

PAEDOPHILIA (SEXUAL ATTRACTION TO CHILDREN)

This may lead to an adult engaging in sexual activity with a child of the same or opposite sex – a criminal offence. Where the child is an older girl (over 12 years of age) the offender tends to be a young male, relatively indiscriminate about sexual partners but neither consistently deviant nor psychiatrically ill. For children below the age of puberty the adult is likely to be substantially older than the child and more consistently interested in sexual activity with children. They are also more likely to have a mental disorder, such as schizophrenia, hypomania, alcohol dependence, dementia or mental handicap (Bancroft, 1989).

TRANSVESTISM

This is defined as persistent wearing of clothes of the opposite sex (cross-dressing). There is a broad range of such behaviour, from the occasional wearing by a man of one female garment to regularly dressing entirely in female clothing. It is usually done by a heterosexual man for the purpose of sexual excitement. Cross-dressing in order to fulfil a social role without sexual excitement is the form taken by transvestism as part of transsexualism (Sims, 1988).

EXHIBITIONISM

In exhibitionism the main sexual expression and gratification are derived from exposure of the genitals to a person of the opposite sex (Snaith, 1983). This leads to the most common sexual offence in the UK (i.e. 'indecent exposure'). There are two types:

1. Type I, which accounts for some 80% of cases. Inhibited young men, emotionally immature, who struggle against the impulse, usually expose a flaccid penis and feel guilty afterwards. They have a good prognosis.

2. Type 2, which accounts for 20% of cases. Men with sociopathic personality who expose the erect penis, often masturbate whilst exposing, show little guilt and may take sadistic pleasure in what they are doing. They have a much worse prognosis (Rooth, 1975).

FETISHISM

Fetishism means 'the worship of inanimate objects', but in a modern sense refers to a repeated sexual preoccupation and excitement with non-living objects, which have a central importance in achieving sexual arousal/orgasm (Sims, 1988). The subject of the fetish may be an article of clothing (such as shoes of the opposite sex), a substance (like rubber) or a texture (such as fur). The fetishistic object may be used in sexual behaviour either alone or involving another person.

VOYEURISM

Voyeurism is the use, to achieve sexual excitement, of viewing unsuspecting people who are naked, undressing or engaged in sexual activity. Masturbation may take place during or after viewing.

FROTTEURISM

Frotteurism involves touching and rubbing against a non-consenting person. This usually occurs in a busy place likely to allow a better chance of avoiding arrest (e.g. a crowded underground train). Whilst rubbing his genitals against the victim's thighs or buttocks, or touching her genitalia or breasts with his hands, the perpetrator may fantasize an exclusive, caring relationship with the victim (American Psychiatric Association, 1994).

SADO-MASOCHISM

Sado–masochism means sexual arousal in response to the infliction of pain, psychological humiliation or ritualized dominance or submission. Sadism is the infliction of pain or suffering upon another for sexual excitement. Masochism is sexual excitement gained from the passive experience of being made to suffer (Sims, 1988).

NECROPHILIA

Necrophilia involves achieving sexual excitement through contact with a dead body. It is very rare and may be associated with murder.

POLYMORPHOUSLY PERVERSE

'Polymorphously perverse' is a phrase used to describe individuals who find sexual excitement and gratification through many different paraphilic behaviours, such as those listed above.

Treatment for paraphilias

Perhaps the most serious of the paraphilias recognized in ICD-10 and DSM-IV which can result in dangerous anti-social behaviour is paedophilia (World Health Organization, 1992; American Psychiatric Association, 1994). There is no well established treatment for this problem, but in some cases, where there is associated hypersexuality, attempts have been made to treat patients with drugs that suppress androgen secretion and so may abolish or reduce sexual drive and desire. Hypersexuality is poorly defined. Sex drive may be low, normal or high (hypersexual), and sexual behaviour may sometimes be compulsive, with or without a paraphilia. Subjects who are hypersexual and have a compulsive element to a dangerous paraphilia obviously pose a particular threat to society; it is towards this group that anti-androgen therapy is particularly directed (Bradford and Pawlak, 1993).

As stated and explained in the introduction to this book, the main focus has been on sexual dysfunction rather than other types of sexual problems such as the paraphilias or gender identity disorders. For a more detailed account of the nature, aetiology and management of paraphilias, the reader is directed to the chapter on *Sexual and Gender Identity Disorders* in DSM-IV (American Psychiatric Association, 1994).

Gender identity disorders

Gender can be manifested in at least seven different ways (Bancroft, 1989):

- Chromosomes
- Gonads
- Hormones
- Internal sexual organs
- External genitalia and secondary sexual characteristics
- Gender assigned at birth ('it's a boy')
- **Gender identity** ('I'm a girl')

Problems of gender identity are largely subsumed within the concept of 'transsexualism'. Transsexual individuals persistently feel an incongruity between their anatomical sex and gender identity. They will tend to complain of a sense that they are "trapped inside the wrong body". Their own gender identity does not match the appearance of their genitals and secondary sexual characteristics (Masters *et al.*, 1995). The biologically male transsexual wishes to change to female anatomy and to live as a woman; and vice versa. The male to female type is much more common than female to male. One estimated prevalence for the former is 1 in 100,000 men (Pauly, 1974).

Gender identity disorders

Gender identity disorder in children
    Specifier:
    • Sexually attracted to males/females/both/neither

Gender identity disorder in adolescents or adults
    Specifier:
    • Sexually attracted to males/females/both/neither

Gender identity disorder NOS
Sexual disorder NOS

TABLE 11. Classifying gender identity disorders. Reprinted with permission from the *Diagnostic and Statistical Manual of Mental Disorders*, fourth edition. Copyright 2000. American Psychiatric Association.

Treatment for gender identity disorders

Psychotherapy alone has been generally unsuccessful in resolving the distress felt by these people as a result of their predicament (Tollinson and Adams, 1979). As a result, services to help such people, possibly with what is often their ultimate and stated goal of gender reassignment (or 'sex change'), require a multi-speciality team approach including psychiatric/ psychological, endocrinological and surgical elements. In view of the irreversible nature of surgical gender reassignment, a cautious approach is taken to offering it. This includes up to a 2-year trial period, during which time the individual is required to live openly as a person of the opposite sex. They will be expected to adopt hairstyles, clothing and mannerisms of that sex and to assume a name that fits with their new gender. If they are able to do all of this they will move on to hormonal and surgical treatment, as required. Varying success rates have been reported, including one paper which provides an overview of 11 different follow-up studies. This concluded that 87% of male to female transsexuals have a 'satisfactory outcome', with this number rising to 97% for female to male cases (Green and Fleming, 1990). With regard to the latter, however, female to male subjects do not necessarily opt for any attempt at surgical construction of a penis.

As stated and explained in the introduction to this book, the main focus has been on sexual dysfunction rather than other types of sexual problems such as the paraphilias or gender identity disorders. For a more detailed account of the nature, aetiology and management of gender identity problems, the reader is directed to the chapter on *Sexual and Gender Identity Disorders* in DSM-IV (American Psychiatric Association, 1994).

References and bibliography

American Psychiatric Association (1994) *Diagnostic and Statistical Manual of Mental Disorders*, fourth revision. APA Press: Washington, DC.

Apfelbaum, B. (2000) Retarded ejaculation: a much misunderstood syndrome. In: Leiblum, S.R. and Rosen, R.C. (eds), *Principles and Practice of Sex Therapy*, third edition. The Guilford Press: London.

Balls, M. (2003) Personal communication.

Balon, R., Yeragani, V.K., Pohl, R. *et al.* (1993) Sexual dysfunction during antidepressant treatment. *J Clin Psychiatry* **54**(6): 209–212.

Bancroft, J. (1989) *Human Sexuality and its Problems*, second edition. Churchill Livingstone: Edinburgh.

Bancroft, J. (1998) Sexual disorders. In: Johnstone, E.C., Lawrie, S., Owens, D. *et al.* (eds), *Companion to Psychiatric Studies*, sixth edition, pp. 529–550. Churchill Livingstone: Edinburgh.

Basson, R. (2001) Female sexual response: the role of drugs in management of sexual dysfunction. *Obstet Gynecol* **98**(2): 350–353.

Basson, R., Berman J., Burnett A. *et al.* (2000) Report of the international consensus development conference on female sexual dysfunction: definitions and classifications. *J Urol* **163**: 888–893.

Bazire, S. (2001) Selecting drugs, doses and preparations – sexual dysfunction. In: *Psychotropic Drug Directory 2001/2002*, pp.165–171. Mark Allen Publishing Ltd: Salisbury.

Beck, A.T. (1967) *Depression: Clinical, Experimental and Theoretical Aspects*. Staples Press: London.

Begg, A., Dickerson, M. and Loudon, N.B. (1976) Frequency of self-reported sexual problems in a family planning clinic. *J Fam Plan Doc* **2**: 41–48.

Bradford, J. and Pawlak, A. (1993) Double-blind placebo cross-over study of cyproterone acetate in the treatment of the paraphilias. *Arch Sex Behav* **22**: 383–402.

British Medical Association (2004) Drugs for erectile dysfunction. In: BNF (British National Formulary), volume 48, pp. 417–420. BMA: London.

Burnap, D.W. and Golden, G.S. (1967) Sexual problems in medical practice. *J Med Ed* **42**: 673–680.

Butcher, J. (1999) Female sexual problems: loss of desire – what about the fun? *BMJ* **318**: 41–43.

Catalan, J., Bradley, M., Gallwey, J. *et al.* (1981) Sexual dysfunction and psychiatric morbidity in patients attending a clinic for sexually transmitted diseases. *Br J Psychiatry* **138**: 292–296.

Cawood, H.H. and Bancroft, J. (1996) Steroid hormones, menopause, sexuality and well-being of women. *Psychol Physiol Med* **26**: 925–936.

Clayton, D.O. and Shen, W.W. (1998) Psychotropic drug-induced sexual function disorders. *Drug Safety* **19**(4): 299–312.

Crowe, M. (1998) Sexual therapy and the couple. In: Freeman, H. (ed.), *Seminars in Psychosexual Disorders*, pp 59–83. Gaskell: London.

Crowe, M. and Jones, M. (1992) Sex therapy: the successes, the failures, the future. *Br J Hosp Med* **48**(8): 474–482.

Crowe, M. and Ridley, J. (2000) *Therapy with Couples*. Blackwell Science: Oxford.

Delvin, D. (1974) *The Book of Love*. New English Library: London.

Drife, J. (2003) Personal communication.

Ellenberg, M. (1977) Sexual aspects of the female diabetic. *Mount Sinai J Med* **44**(4): 495–500.

Feldman, H., Goldstein, I., Hatzichristou, D.G. *et al.* (1994) Impotence and its medical and psychosocial correlates: results of the Massachusetts male ageing study. *J Urol* **151**(1): 54–61.

Frank, E., Anderson, C. and Rubenstein, D. (1978) Frequency of sexual dysfunction in 'normal' couples. *NEJM* **299**: 111–115.

Gebhard, P.H. (1978) Marital stress. In: Lev, L. (ed.), *Society, Stress and Disease, Volume 3: The Productive and Reproductive Age*. Oxford University Press: Oxford.

Gebhard, P.H. and Johnson, A.B. (1979) *Kinsey Data: marginal tabulations of the 1938–1963 interviews conducted by the Institute for Sex Research*. Saunders: Philadelphia.

Goldberg, D.C., Whipple, B., Fishkin, R.E. *et al.* (1983) The Grafenberg spot and female ejaculation: a review of initial hypotheses. *J Sex Marital Ther* **9**: 27–37.

Gordon, P. (1994) The contribution of sexology to contemporary sexuality education. *J Sex Marital Ther* **9**(2): 171–180.

Green, R. and Fleming, D.T. (1990) Transsexual surgery follow-up: status in the 1990s. *Ann Rev Sex Res* **1**: 163–174.

Hawton, K. (1982) The behavioural treatment of sexual dysfunction. *Br J Psychiatry* **140**: 94–101.

Hawton, K. (1984) Sexual adjustment of men who have had strokes. *J Psychosom Res* **28**: 243–249.

Hawton, K. (1985) *Sex Therapy: A Practical Guide*. Oxford University Press: Oxford.

Hawton, K. and Catalan, J. (1986) Prognostic factors in sex therapy. *Behav Res Ther* **24**(4): 377–385.

Hawton, K., Catalan, J., Martin, M. *et al.* (1986) Long-term outcome of sex therapy. *Behav Res Ther* **24**(6): 665–675.

Heiman, J.R. and LoPiccolo, J. (1999) *Becoming Orgasmic*, second edition. Piatkus: London.

Heiman, J.R., Quirk, F.H., Rosen, R.C. *et al.* (2002) Development of a sexual function questionnaire for clinical trials of female sexual dysfunction. *J Wom Health Gender-Based Med* **11**(3): 277–289.

Hetherington, E.M. and Stanley-Hagan, M. (1999) The adjustment of children with divorced parents: a risk and resiliency perspective. *J Child Psychol Psychiatry* **40**(1): 129–140.

Holland, A.R. (2002) An evaluation of assessment and outcome tools used by psychosexual therapists across the UK. MSc dissertation, University of Central Lancashire.

Howard, P. and Allwood, D. (2002) Erectile dysfunction prescription maintenance scheme in Leeds Teaching Hospitals NHS Trust. Personal communication.

Hunt, M. (1975) *Sexual Behaviour in the 1970s*. Dell: New York.

Hutchison, T.A., Shahan, D.R. and Anderson, M.L. (2002) (eds) *Drugdex System, Internet Version*. Micromedex Inc: Colorado [4.3.02].

Impotence Association (1997) *Key Findings of the Impotence Association Patient and Partner Erectile Dysfunction Survey 1997*. Impotence Association: London.

Kaplan, H.S. (1989) *PE: How to Overcome Premature Ejaculation*. Brunner/Mazel: New York.

Kinsey, A.C., Pomeroy, W.B. and Martin, C.E. (1948) *Sexual Behaviour in the Human Male*. Saunders: Philadelphia.

Kinsey, A.C., Pomeroy, W.B., Martin, C.E. *et al*. (1953) *Sexual Behaviour in the Human Female*. Saunders: Philadelphia.

Kurt, U., Ozkardes, H., Altug, U. *et al*. (1994) The efficacy of anti-serotonergic agents in the treatment of erectile dysfunction. *J Urol* **152**(2): 407–409.

Ladas, A.K., Whipple, B. and Perry, J.D. (1982) *The G Spot and Other Recent Discoveries about Human Sexuality*. Holt, Rinehart and Winston: New York.

Laumann, E.O., Paik, A. and Rosen, R.C. (1999) Sexual dysfunction in the United States: prevalence and predictors. *JAMA* **10**: 537–545.

Levine, S.B. and Yost, M.A. (1976) Frequency of sexual dysfunction in a general gynaecological clinic: an epidemiological approach. *Arch Sex Behav* **5**: 229–238.

Lilius, H.G., Valtonen, E.J. and Wilkstrom, J. (1976) Sexual problems in patients suffering from multiple sclerosis. *J Chronic Dis* **29**: 643–647.

Ludovico, G.M, Corvasce, A., Pagliarulo, G. *et al*. (1996) Paroxetine in the treatment of premature ejaculation. *Br J Urol* **77**: 881–882.

Maguire, G.P., Lee, E.G., Bevington, D.J. *et al*. (1978) Psychiatric problems in the first year after mastectomy. *BMJ* **1**: 963–965.

Masters, W.H. and Johnson, V.E. (1966) *Human Sexual Response*. Churchill: London.

Masters, W.H. and Johnson, V.E. (1970) *Human Sexual Inadequacy*. Churchill: London.

Masters, W.H., Johnson, V.E. and Kolodny, R.C. (1995) *Human Sexuality*, fifth edition. Harper Collins: New York.

Mathew, R.J. and Weinman, M.L. (1982) Sexual dysfunction in depression. *Arch Sex Behav* **11**: 323–328.

McCulloch, D.K., Campbell, I.W., Wu, F.C. *et al*. (1980) The prevalence of diabetic impotence. *Diabetologia* **18**: 279–283.

Medicines Control Agency (2002) Reminder: use of traditional Chinese medicines and herbal remedies. *Curr Prob Pharmacovigilance* **28**: 6.

Morales, A. (2001) Apomorphine to Uprima: the development of a practical erectogenic drug: a personal perspective. *Int J Impot Res* **13**(Suppl. 3): 29–34.

O'Connor, T.G., Thorpe, K., Dunn, J. *et al*. (1999) Parental divorce and adjustment in adulthood: findings from a community sample. *J Child Psychol Psychiatry* **40**(5): 777–789.

Pauly, I.B. (1974) Female transsexualism: part I. *Arch Sex Behav* **3:** 487–507.

Pfizer Global Research and Development (1997) *The Female Sexual Functioning Questionnaire (SFQ)*. Pfizer: Manchester.

Ralph, D. and McNicholas, T. (2000) UK management guidelines for erectile dysfunction. *BMJ* **321:** 499–503.

Riley, A. (1999) *Sexual Drive (Libido) Disorders*. Presentation at: 'First International Conference on Sexual Disorders', Royal College of Physicians, London.

Rooth, F.G. (1975) Indecent exposure and exhibitionism. *Br J Psychiatry* **Spec No 9:** 212–222.

Rosen, R.C., Riley, A., Wagner, G. *et al.* (1997) The international index of erectile function (IIEF): a multidimensional scale for assessment of erectile dysfunction. *Urology* **49**(6): 822–830.

Royal College of Psychiatrists (2001) *Curriculum for Basic Specialist Training and the MRCPsych Examination (CR95).* Gaskell: London.

Rubin, A. and Babbott, D. (1958) Impotence and diabetes mellitus. *JAMA* **168**: 498–500.

Rust, J., Bennun, I., Crowe, M. *et al.* (1988) The Golombok Rust Inventory of Marital State (GRIMS). nfer-NELSON: Windsor.

Segraves, R.T. (1988) Sexual side-effects of psychiatric drugs. *Int J Psychiat Med* **18:** 243–252.

Selvini Palazolli, M., Boscolo, L., Cecchin, G. *et al.* (1978) *Paradox and Counter-Paradox.* Jason Aronson: New York.

Sims, A.C.P. (1988) *Symptoms in the Mind: An Introduction to Descriptive Psychopathology.* Balliere Tindall: London.

Snaith, R.P. (1983) Exhibitionism: a clinical conundrum. *Br J Psychiatry* **143:** 231–235.

Snell, R.S. (1981) *Clinical Anatomy for Medical Students.* Little, Brown and Company: Boston.

Stein, G. (1995) Drug treatment of the personality disorders, premenstrual tension, impotence and male sexual suppressants. In: King, D. (ed.), *Seminars in Clinical Psychopharmacology.* Gaskell: London.

Swan, M. and Wilson, L.J. (1979) Sexual and marital problems in a psychiatric out-patient population. *Br J Psychiatry* **135**: 310–314.

Tavris, C. and Sadd, S. (1977) *The Redbook Report on Female Sexuality.* Delacorte Press: New York.

Taylor, D., Duncan, D., Mir, S. *et al.* (1997) Antidepressant-induced sexual dysfunction: new antidepressants. *Drug Inform Quart* **4**(2): 6–9.

Tollinson, C.D. and Adams, H.E. (1979) *Sexual Disorders: Treatment, Theory, Research.* Gardner Press: New York.

Trigwell, P.J., Yates, A.F.J. and Coburn, S.A. (2004) *Database of the Leeds Psychosexual Medicine Service: The First 1000 Referrals,* in preparation.

Vas, C.J. (1978) Sexual impotence and some autonomic disturbances in men with multiple sclerosis. In: Comfort, A. (ed.), *Sexual Consequences of Disability,* pp. 45–60. Stickley: Philadelphia.

Virag, R., Bouilly, P. and Frydman, D. (1985) Is impotence an arterial disorder? A study of arterial risk factors in 440 impotent men. *Lancet* **1**: 181–184.

Wadsworth, M.E.J. (1986) Grounds for divorce in England and Wales: a social and demographic analysis. *J Biosoc Sci* **18**: 127–153.

Wagner, G. and Metz, P. (1981) Arteriosclerosis and erectile failure. In: Wagner, G. and Green, R. (eds), *Impotence: Physiological, Surgical Diagnosis and Treatment.* Plenum: New York.

Waldinger, M.D., Hengeveld, M.W. and Zwinderman, A.H. (1994) Paroxetine treatment of premature ejaculation: a double-blind, randomized, placebo-controlled study. *Am J Psychiatry* **151**(9): 1377–1379.

World Health Organization (1992) *The ICD-10 Classification of Mental and Behavioural Disorders: Clinical Descriptions and Diagnostic Guidelines.* World Health Organization: Geneva.

Zilbergeld, B. (1978) *Men and Sex.* Harper Collins: London.

Appendix: how to acquire useful resources

When helping people with sexual problems, clinicians often find it useful to be able to suggest various resources to their patient(s). These may include books, lubricants, vaginal trainers, or items to help the person or couple to maximize their sexual arousal. The following is a list of addresses through which such resources are available at the time of writing this book. This is by no means an exhaustive list. It simply represents companies which the author and his colleagues have found are easy to use, discreet and reliable. Most are website addresses or telephone numbers because many people find it more acceptable and easier to buy products such as these by internet or phone rather than at a 'high street' shop.

Abbey Books (for '*How to Overcome Premature Ejaculation*' and other self-help books)
- +44 (0)1332 290021

Amielle (for vaginal trainers for use in treating vaginismus)
- +44 (0)800 7316959: for patients to order trainers
- +44 (0)1993 810052: for clinicians to obtain further information

Ann Summers (for a range of sex aids, clothing, etc.)
- www.annsummers.com
- +44 (0)845 4562399
- Also stores in many UK towns and cities

Emotional Bliss (for a modern and sophisticated range of vibrators)
- www.emotionalbliss.co.uk
- +44 (0)870 0410022

LTC Healthcare/The Leeds Trading Co. (for condoms, lubricants, vibrators, etc.)
- www.cw4play.com
- +44 (0)1423 815550

Sex Ware Catalogue (for vibrators, other sex aids, instructional
adult videos, etc.)
- www.fpsales.co.uk
- +44 (0)870 4445116

Sexual Dysfunction Association (for information, e.g. leaflets, and
support)
- www.sda.uk.net
- +44 (0)870 7743571

Vacuum pumps (indicated in some cases of erectile dysfunction)
- Osbon Erecaid: info@osbonmedical.co.uk
                    +44 (0)845 6588877
- SomaErect: Imedicare@aol.com
                    +44 (0)20 82075627
- Rapport: +44 (0)1993 810052 for information
                    +44 (0)800 7316959 to order

Index

Notes
All index entries refer to sexual problems, unless otherwise indicated.
Page numbers followed by 'f' indicate figures; page numbers followed by 't' indicate tables.